CKD STAGE 3 A

TYPE 2 COOKBOOK FOR

SENIORS

A comprehensive guide with tasty and nutritious kidney friendly and diabetes diet recipes.

Olivia Endwell

Copyright Statement:

Disclaimer:

The information provided in this book is for educational and informational purposes only. It is not intended as a substitute for professional medical advice, diagnosis, or treatment. Always seek the advice of your physician or other qualified health provider with any questions you may have regarding a medical condition. Never disregard professional medical advice or delay in seeking it because of something you have read in this book.

The author and publisher disclaim any liability arising directly or indirectly from the use of this book. The information provided is based on the author's best knowledge at the time of writing and is subject to change. The author and publisher do not guarantee the accuracy, completeness, or timeliness of the information presented in this book.

TABLE OF CONTENTS

INTRODUCTION

Hey there! So, we're diving into the world of chronic kidney disease (CKD) Stage 3 and Diabetes Type 2 – two health buzzwords that might sound a bit overwhelming, especially for our seniors. But don't worry, we're here to break it down and make it as clear as day.

Let's kick things off with CKD Stage 3. Picture your kidneys as superheroes in your body, filtering out the bad stuff. Now, when they hit Stage 3, it's like they've been in a bit of a battle – some damage, but they're still hanging in there. That's where we step in with lifestyle changes, a kidney-friendly diet, and keeping a close eye on things to keep those kidneys kicking.

Now, onto Diabetes Type 2, the blood sugar tango. It's like a dance where insulin is the star, but sometimes it gets a bit shy. We'll chat about how the body handles sugar, why it sometimes plays hard to get, and how we can keep things groovy with lifestyle tweaks and maybe a bit of medication magic.

So, here's the deal: We want you to understand the nitty-gritty of these conditions because knowledge is power. We're not here to bog you down with medical jargon; we're here to chat about how your body works, why these conditions happen, and what we can do about it.

Throughout this cookbook, we'll sprinkle in practical tips, easy-to-follow advice, and some darn delicious recipes to help you take charge of your health. It's all about finding that sweet spot (pun intended!) where good food meets good health, making your journey through CKD Stage 3 and Diabetes Type 2 a bit more manageable and a whole lot tastier. Let's get started on this health and flavor adventure together!

CHAPTER 1: MANAGING DIET FOR CKD AND DIABETES

Dietary Guidelines for CKD Stage 3 and Diabetes Type 2

Navigating the dietary landscape when you're dealing with both Chronic Kidney Disease (CKD) Stage 3 and Diabetes Type 2 requires a strategic approach. It's like crafting a personalized roadmap for your meals, one that addresses the unique challenges of these conditions. Let's break it down.

First off, CKD Stage 3. At this stage, your kidneys are putting up a fight, but they need a bit of extra TLC. Enter dietary guidelines tailored to support kidney health. We're talking about moderating protein intake, keeping a close eye on phosphorus and potassium levels, and managing fluid intake. It's a delicate balance that aims to ease the workload on your kidneys while ensuring you still get the nutrients you need.

Now, throw Diabetes Type 2 into the mix. Blood sugar management becomes a key player in our dietary strategy. We're looking at controlling carbohydrates, understanding the glycemic index, and maintaining steady blood sugar levels throughout the day. It's a bit of a juggling act, but with the right knowledge, it can be a well-choreographed dance.

So, how do we merge these two sets of guidelines into a cohesive plan? It involves smart food choices, portion control, and a dash of creativity in the kitchen. Throughout this chapter, we'll explore practical tips and tasty recipes that align with these dietary guidelines, offering a helping hand in managing both CKD Stage 3 and Diabetes Type 2 through the power of nutrition.

Balancing Carbohydrates, Proteins, and Fats

Let's dive into the macronutrient trio: carbohydrates, proteins, and fats. Balancing these components is like tuning an instrument – get it just right, and the symphony (or in this case, your health) flourishes.

Carbohydrates: When it comes to Diabetes Type 2, keeping an eye on your carbohydrate intake is crucial. Not all carbs are created equal, and understanding the difference between complex and simple carbs can make a world of difference. We'll explore the concept of the glycemic index, helping you choose carbs that won't send your blood sugar on a rollercoaster ride.

Proteins: For CKD Stage 3, protein becomes a bit of a tricky character. On one hand, you need it for muscle health and overall well-being. On the other, too much can put strain on your kidneys. We'll unravel the protein mystery, discussing high-quality sources and how to strike the right balance for kidney-friendly meals that still pack a protein punch.

Fats: Not all fats are villains; some are downright heroes. We'll chat about the good fats – unsaturated fats that support heart health – and the not-so-friendly saturated fats that may need a bit of moderation. Balancing fats is not just about quantity but also about choosing the right sources to benefit both your heart and kidneys.

By the end of this exploration, you'll have a solid understanding of how to create a macronutrient harmony that caters to the intricacies of CKD Stage 3 and Diabetes Type 2, making every bite a step toward better health.

Importance of Fiber in the Diet

Picture fiber as the unsung hero of your meals – not flashy but absolutely crucial for your well-being. And when you're dealing with CKD Stage 3 and Diabetes Type 2, fiber takes on an even more significant role.

Fiber is like the janitor of your digestive system, sweeping away unwanted elements and keeping things moving smoothly. For individuals with Diabetes Type 2, fiber becomes a blood sugar superhero. It slows down the absorption of sugar, preventing those pesky spikes and crashes. And for those with CKD Stage 3, a high-fiber diet can help control blood pressure and improve overall gut health.

In this section, we'll explore the two types of fiber – soluble and insoluble – and how they contribute to your well-being. We'll also delve into delicious and fiber-rich foods, offering practical tips on incorporating them into your daily meals. From whole grains to colorful veggies and legumes, fiber is the unsung hero you'll want on your plate every day.

Understanding the role of fiber in the diet isn't just about ticking off a nutritional checklist; it's about embracing a lifestyle that supports your digestive health, blood sugar management, and overall vitality.

Monitoring Sodium Intake

Ah, the sneaky culprit in many modern diets – sodium. For individuals grappling with both CKD Stage 3 and Diabetes Type 2, keeping an eye on sodium intake becomes a crucial aspect of dietary management.

Sodium has a way of hiding in plain sight, often in processed foods, condiments, and restaurant dishes. For those with CKD Stage 3, excess sodium can contribute to fluid retention and increased blood pressure, putting additional strain on already compromised kidneys. Meanwhile, individuals with Diabetes Type 2 need to be cautious as high sodium levels can impact blood pressure, potentially leading to cardiovascular complications.

In this section, we'll embark on a sodium exploration – understanding where it lurks, decoding food labels, and discovering flavorful alternatives. We'll also discuss the delicate art of seasoning without overloading on sodium, empowering you to take control of your salt intake without sacrificing taste.

By the end of this journey, you'll be equipped with the knowledge and practical tips needed to navigate the sodium landscape, ensuring your meals are not only delicious but also supportive of both your kidney and blood sugar health.

CHAPTER 2: MONITORING AND MANAGING HEALTH

Regular Health Checkups and Monitoring

Alright, let's kick off our health journey with a topic that's often underestimated but packs a powerful punch – regular health checkups and monitoring. Picture it as giving your body a tune-up, a chance to catch any potential hiccups before they turn into full-blown symphonies of health issues.

When you're dealing with Chronic Kidney Disease (CKD) Stage 3 and Diabetes Type 2, these regular checkups become your superhero cape, helping you stay one step ahead of any twists and turns in your health story. But what exactly does a health checkup involve, and why is it crucial?

A regular health checkup isn't just a quick visit to the doctor's office; it's a comprehensive assessment of your overall well-being. Your healthcare team will likely check your blood pressure, monitor your weight, and assess your blood and urine samples. These routine measurements can provide valuable insights into the state of your kidneys and blood sugar levels.

For CKD Stage 3, monitoring becomes especially vital. Regular checkups allow healthcare professionals to track changes in your kidney function, detect any signs of complications, and adjust your treatment plan accordingly. It's like having a roadmap for your health journey – the more checkpoints you have, the better you can navigate the terrain.

In the realm of Diabetes Type 2, regular monitoring is the key to successful blood sugar management. Checking your blood sugar levels regularly empowers you to understand how your body responds to different foods, activities, and medications. It's not just about the numbers on the glucose meter; it's about gaining insights into your unique body rhythms and making informed decisions to keep your blood sugar in check.

Think of these checkups as preventive measures, catching issues while they're still in the minor leagues. Early detection allows for early intervention, potentially preventing complications and ensuring you're on the right track for a healthier tomorrow.

But hey, it's not just about the physical aspects of health. These checkups are also an opportunity to have open and honest conversations with your healthcare team. Discussing any concerns, asking questions about your treatment plan, and sharing how you're feeling can strengthen the bond between you and your healthcare provider. It's a partnership, and you're at the forefront of your health journey.

So, don't skip those checkups! Consider them as your health pit stops, where you refuel with information, make adjustments to your health vehicle, and ensure you're on the smoothest route to well-being.

Blood Sugar Monitoring

Now, let's zoom in on a crucial aspect of managing Diabetes Type 2 – blood sugar monitoring. It's like keeping tabs on your body's financial health, checking in regularly to make sure everything is in balance.

For individuals with Diabetes Type 2, blood sugar levels are the heartbeats of their health story. Monitoring these levels isn't just a routine; it's a lifeline. But why is it so crucial, and how does it play a starring role in your health narrative?

Firstly, let's understand what blood sugar is and why it needs a watchful eye. Blood sugar, or glucose, is the main source of energy for your body's cells. However, when you have Diabetes Type 2, your body struggles to use insulin effectively, leading to elevated blood sugar levels. Monitoring these levels allows you to catch any spikes or dips, preventing potential complications.

Think of blood sugar monitoring as your personal detective work. You're on the lookout for patterns, clues that reveal how your body reacts to different foods, activities, and medications. Is that bowl of pasta sending your blood sugar on a rollercoaster ride? Does a morning walk help keep your levels steady? These are the mysteries you're solving with each blood sugar check.

Now, let's talk tools – the glucose meter, a small but mighty device. It's your sidekick in this journey, providing real-time feedback on your blood sugar levels. Some meters even come with fancy features like trend tracking and mealtime markers, making your detective work a bit more high-tech.

Consistency is the key here. Regular blood sugar monitoring gives you a comprehensive view of your diabetes management. It allows you and your healthcare team to make informed decisions about your treatment plan, lifestyle adjustments, and potential medication changes.

But beyond the numbers, blood sugar monitoring is also about tuning in to your body. How do you feel when your levels are within the target range? Are there symptoms that pop up when they're a bit off track? By connecting the dots between your blood sugar levels and your everyday experiences, you become the author of your health story.

Remember, blood sugar monitoring is not just about managing diabetes; it's about living well with diabetes. Embrace it as a tool for empowerment, a way to take charge of your health narrative, and a means to ensure each chapter is filled with vitality.

Understanding Kidney Function Tests

Now, let's dive into the world of kidneys and understanding kidney function tests. It's like peeking under the hood of your car to see how the engine is running – an essential check to ensure everything is in tip-top shape.

For those dealing with Chronic Kidney Disease (CKD) Stage 3, these tests become your health compass, guiding your healthcare team in understanding how well your kidneys are functioning. But why are they necessary, and what do these tests reveal about your kidney health?

Kidney function tests are a series of blood and urine tests that provide valuable insights into how well your kidneys are filtering waste and maintaining the balance of essential substances in your body. These tests measure key markers, such as creatinine and blood urea nitrogen (BUN), to assess your kidney function.

Creatinine, a waste product produced by muscles, is normally filtered out by the kidneys. Elevated levels in the blood can indicate reduced kidney function. Meanwhile, BUN measures the amount of nitrogen in the blood that comes from urea, a byproduct of protein metabolism. An increase in BUN levels may suggest impaired kidney function.

But understanding these numbers is not just about decoding a series of mysterious digits. It's about comprehending what they mean for your overall health. Your healthcare team will interpret these results, considering your age, sex, and other factors to tailor a treatment plan that suits your unique needs.

Regular kidney function tests are like health check-ins for your kidneys. They allow your healthcare team to monitor any changes in your kidney function over time, providing an early warning system for potential complications. Catching issues in the early stages gives you a head start in implementing lifestyle changes, adjusting your diet, and fine-tuning your treatment plan.

For those in the CKD Stage 3 arena, these tests play a starring role in determining the progression of kidney disease. They help assess whether your kidneys are holding steady, experiencing a slowdown in function, or needing a bit more support.

Beyond the clinical aspect, understanding kidney function tests is about being an active participant in your health journey. Ask questions, seek explanations, and be curious about how these tests contribute to your well-being. Knowledge is power, and when it comes to your kidneys, being informed is your greatest asset.

Medication Management

Now, let's chat about a crucial element in the management of Chronic Kidney Disease (CKD) Stage 3 and Diabetes Type 2 – medication management. It's like conducting a well-orchestrated symphony, with each medication playing a specific role in keeping your health melody in harmony.

When you're dealing with these health challenges, medications often become integral to your treatment plan. But understanding the what, why, and how of your medications is essential for effective management and optimal well-being.

Let's start with the basics – why medications? For CKD Stage 3, medications may be prescribed to manage blood pressure, regulate electrolyte levels, and control conditions that could impact kidney function. Diabetes Type 2 often involves medications to improve insulin sensitivity, lower blood sugar levels, and reduce the risk of complications.

Now, let's debunk a common misconception – medication is not a one-size-fits-all solution. Your healthcare team will tailor your medication plan based on your specific health profile, considering factors such as age, overall health, and the progression of your conditions.

Understanding your medications involves more than just popping pills; it's about becoming a proactive player in your health narrative. Here's a quick rundown of key aspects to consider:

1. Know Your Medications: Familiarize yourself with the names, purposes, and potential side effects of your medications. It's like knowing the characters in your health story.

2. Follow the Prescription: Stick to the prescribed dosage and schedule. Consistency is key in ensuring your medications work optimally.

3. Communicate with Your Healthcare Team: If you experience any side effects or have concerns about your medications, don't hesitate to communicate with your healthcare provider. They can adjust your treatment plan or explore alternative options.

4. Be Aware of Interactions: Some medications may interact with others or with certain foods. Understanding these interactions can prevent potential complications.

5. Regular Check-Ins: Schedule regular follow-ups with your healthcare team to assess the effectiveness of your medications, make adjustments as needed, and address any concerns.

Medication management is not a passive role; it's about being an engaged and informed participant in your health journey. It's acknowledging that medications are tools in your wellness toolkit, working in tandem with lifestyle adjustments, dietary changes, and other aspects of your treatment plan.

Beyond the technicalities, medication management is about embracing a holistic approach to health. It's understanding that medications are one facet of your well-being, and their effectiveness is amplified when combined with a healthy lifestyle, regular monitoring, and open communication with your healthcare team.

So, whether it's a pill, an injection, or a routine checkup, each element of medication management contributes to the symphony of your health. Embrace it as a collaborative effort between you and your healthcare team, where the goal is not just managing conditions but thriving in your journey toward optimal well-being.

CHAPTER 3: KITCHEN TIPS AND TRICKS

Smart Cooking Techniques for Seniors

Cooking is not just a chore; it's an art, a delightful journey that leads to a plate of nourishment and satisfaction. However, for seniors navigating the kitchen, it might sometimes feel like a daunting task. Fear not, for this section is all about smart cooking techniques tailored to make the culinary journey not only manageable but enjoyable.

As we age, certain physical changes might influence how we approach cooking. Reduced strength, dexterity, and energy levels can pose challenges, but with the right techniques, the kitchen can remain a place of creativity and joy.

1. **Ergonomics in the Kitchen:** Start by making your kitchen setup senior-friendly. Arrange frequently used items within easy reach, opt for lightweight cookware, and consider tools with ergonomic handles for a comfortable grip. A well-organized kitchen minimizes unnecessary movements and enhances the overall cooking experience.

2. **One-Pot Wonders:** Embrace the magic of one-pot meals. These dishes not only simplify cooking but also reduce the number of utensils and pots to clean. Whether it's a hearty

stew, a flavorful soup, or a simple stir-fry, one-pot wonders are a time-saving and convenient option for seniors.

3. **Slow Cooker and Instant Pot Magic:** These kitchen gadgets are culinary game-changers. The slow cooker allows you to toss in ingredients in the morning and come back to a fully cooked, delicious meal in the evening. Meanwhile, the Instant Pot can speed up the cooking process without compromising on flavor. Both are excellent choices for seniors looking to simplify their cooking routine.

4. **Prepping Ahead:** Consider doing some prepping in advance to make cooking during the week a breeze. Chop vegetables, marinate proteins, or even prepare entire meals that can be refrigerated or frozen. Having ingredients ready to go reduces the time and effort required for day-to-day cooking.

5. **Easy-to-Use Kitchen Tools:** Invest in kitchen tools designed for ease of use. Look for gadgets with large, easy-to-read dials, non-slip grips, and simple functionalities. From can openers to peelers, having user-friendly tools can significantly enhance the cooking experience.

6. **Adapted Cooking Techniques:** Explore cooking techniques that require less physical effort. For instance, consider using a food processor for chopping and slicing instead of a knife. Opt for cooking methods like baking or steaming that are less hands-on but still produce delicious and nutritious meals.

Remember, the kitchen should be a space of joy, not stress. By incorporating these smart cooking techniques, seniors can continue to enjoy the pleasures of creating and savoring homemade meals without feeling overwhelmed.

Easy Meal Prep Ideas

Meal preparation doesn't have to be a time-consuming or complicated affair. In fact, with a bit of planning and some clever tricks, preparing meals can become a streamlined and enjoyable process. This section is all about easy meal prep ideas that suit the lifestyles of seniors, making the kitchen a place of convenience rather than chaos.

1. **Weekly Meal Planning:** Kickstart your meal prep journey with a weekly meal plan. Outline your meals for the upcoming week, considering variety and nutritional balance. This not only helps with grocery shopping but also provides a roadmap for your daily cooking adventures.

2. **Batch Ingredient Prep:** Take advantage of batch prepping ingredients that can be used in various dishes throughout the week. Chop vegetables, cook grains, or marinate proteins in bulk. Having these basics ready to go significantly cuts down on daily cooking time.

3. **Freezer-Friendly Meals:** Explore recipes that lend themselves well to freezing. Prepare large batches of soups,

stews, casseroles, or sauces, and portion them into individual servings. These frozen meals can be easily reheated for quick and convenient dinners, reducing the need for daily cooking.

4. **Cook Once, Eat Twice:** Opt for meals that can be repurposed for another day. For example, roast a whole chicken for dinner, and then use the leftovers for sandwiches, salads, or a quick stir-fry. This strategy minimizes waste and maximizes the utility of your cooking efforts.

5. **No-Cook Meal Options:** Not every meal requires extensive cooking. Embrace simple, no-cook options like salads, sandwiches, or wraps. These meals not only save time in the kitchen but also provide a refreshing break from the stove.

6. **Portion Control:** Consider portioning out meals in advance. Use containers to divide larger batches into individual servings. This not only makes it easy to grab a meal whenever you're hungry but also helps with maintaining a balanced and controlled diet.

7. **Utilize Convenience Foods:** Don't shy away from utilizing convenient, healthy options. Pre-cut vegetables, canned beans, and frozen fruits can be valuable allies in the kitchen. They save prep time without compromising on nutritional value.

8. **Mix and Match Ingredients:** Create a versatile pantry with staple ingredients that can be mixed and matched in various

ways. A can of beans, for example, can be used in salads, soups, or wraps, providing flexibility and variety in your meals.

The goal of easy meal prep is to simplify the cooking process, allowing seniors to enjoy delicious, homemade meals without spending excessive time or effort in the kitchen. By incorporating these ideas, meal prep becomes a manageable and rewarding aspect of daily life.

Cooking for One or Two

Cooking for smaller households doesn't mean sacrificing variety or flavor. In fact, it opens up opportunities for creativity and exploration in the kitchen. This section focuses on cooking for one or two, providing tips and ideas tailored to the unique needs of smaller households.

1. **Portion Control and Scaling Recipes:** Adjusting recipes for smaller portions is a skill that streamlines cooking for one or two. Learn to scale down ingredient quantities while maintaining the right balance of flavors. This not only reduces waste but also ensures that you're preparing the right amount for your needs.

2. **Embrace Leftovers Creatively:** Leftovers are your kitchen allies. Get creative with repurposing them into new dishes. For instance, yesterday's roasted vegetables can become a

tasty omelet filling, and that grilled chicken can be reinvented as a flavorful sandwich.

3. **Explore Single-Serve Recipes:** Many recipes can be adapted for single servings. Invest time in discovering or creating recipes that suit your preferences and can be easily adjusted for smaller quantities. From desserts to main dishes, single-serve recipes offer variety without excess.

4. **Diversify Cooking Techniques:** Experiment with different cooking techniques that suit smaller portions. For example, consider using smaller kitchen appliances like toaster ovens or countertop grills. These tools are efficient for cooking smaller quantities and can add versatility to your culinary repertoire.

5. **Utilize Pre-Packaged Ingredients:** Leverage pre-packaged ingredients strategically. Pre-packaged salads, pre-cut vegetables, and individually portioned items can be convenient for smaller households. These items reduce prep time and minimize the need for extensive cooking.

6. **Freeze Smartly:** While freezing leftovers is a great option, freezing raw ingredients can also be a game-changer. Portion out items like meat, fruits, or even prepared sauces and freeze them for later use. This ensures you always have a variety of options without the pressure to consume everything immediately.

7. **Invest in Versatile Ingredients:** Stock your pantry with versatile ingredients that can be used in multiple dishes. Items like pasta, rice, canned tomatoes, and various spices can form the foundation of diverse and flavorful meals for one or two.

8. **Plan for Variety:** Just because you're cooking for fewer people doesn't mean your meals have to lack variety. Plan your weekly meals to include different cuisines, flavors, and textures. This approach keeps your culinary experience exciting and enjoyable.

Cooking for one or two is an opportunity to savor the pleasure of creating and enjoying meals without the constraints of larger quantities. By adopting these strategies, smaller households can relish the freedom and creativity that comes with tailoring the kitchen experience to their unique needs.

Batch Cooking for Convenience

Batch cooking is the superhero of time-saving strategies in the kitchen. It's about preparing larger quantities of meals at once and then freezing or refrigerating portions for later use. For seniors managing Chronic Kidney Disease (CKD) Stage 3 and Diabetes Type 2, batch cooking can be a game-changer, providing convenience, variety, and nutritional control.

1. **Planning and Organization:** The key to successful batch cooking is planning. Create a weekly meal plan, identify recipes suitable for batch cooking, and make a comprehensive shopping list. This sets the stage for an organized and efficient cooking session.

2. **Choose Freezer-Friendly Recipes:** Not all recipes are created equal when it comes to batch cooking. Opt for dishes that freeze well without compromising taste or texture. Soups, stews, casseroles, and certain pasta dishes are excellent candidates for batch cooking.

3. **Invest in Storage Containers:** Arm yourself with a variety of storage containers suitable for freezing. Choose containers that are freezer-safe, airtight, and easy to stack. Label each container with the name of the dish and the date of preparation for easy identification.

4. **Portion Control:** While the aim is to prepare larger quantities, it's crucial to maintain portion control. Divide the batch into individual or family-sized portions before freezing. This not only makes it easy to grab a meal when needed but also helps in managing portion sizes.

5. **Variety in Batch Cooking:** Batch cooking doesn't mean monotony. Prepare a variety of dishes to ensure a diverse and exciting menu throughout the week. Rotate between different proteins, grains, and vegetables to keep your meals interesting and nutritionally balanced.

6. **Cook Once, Eat Multiple Times:** Batch cooking allows you to cook once and enjoy the fruits of your labor multiple times. It minimizes the frequency of cooking sessions while providing a steady supply of homemade, nutritious meals.

7. **Time-Saving Cooking Techniques:** Opt for time-saving cooking techniques that are conducive to batch cooking. Slow cooking, roasting, and using the Instant Pot can be particularly efficient when preparing larger quantities.

8. **Adapt Recipes for Dietary Needs:** Batch cooking is customizable to meet specific dietary needs. For those managing CKD Stage 3, pay attention to phosphorus and potassium content in recipes. Similarly, individuals with Diabetes Type 2 can adjust recipes to control carbohydrate intake.

9. **Themed Batch Cooking Days:** Consider organizing themed batch cooking days. For instance, designate a day for preparing proteins, another for grains and legumes, and a third for sauces and soups. This structured approach streamlines the process and ensures a well-rounded menu.

10. **Utilize Batch Cooking for Snacks:** Extend batch cooking to snacks and sides. Prepare items like energy bars, muffins, or roasted vegetables in larger quantities and freeze them for quick and convenient snacks.

Batch cooking empowers seniors to take control of their nutritional intake while minimizing the time and effort spent in the kitchen. It's a practical approach that aligns with the unique needs of individuals managing health conditions, offering a balance between convenience and culinary enjoyment.

CHAPTER 4: BREAKFAST RECIPES

1. Vegetable Omelette with Avocado Toast

Prep Time: 10 minutes

Cooking Time: 10 minutes

Serving Size: 1

Ingredients:

- 2 large eggs

- 1/4 cup diced bell peppers

- 1/4 cup diced tomatoes

- 1/4 cup chopped spinach

- Salt and pepper to taste

- 1 teaspoon olive oil

- 1 slice whole-grain bread

- 1/2 ripe avocado

Instructions:

1. In a bowl, whisk eggs and season with salt and pepper.

2. Heat olive oil in a non-stick pan over medium heat.

3. Add bell peppers, tomatoes, and spinach to the pan. Cook for 2-3 minutes until veggies are slightly tender.

4. Pour the whisked eggs over the vegetables, cook until set, then flip to cook the other side.

5. Toast the whole-grain bread and mash the avocado on top.

6. Serve the omelette on the avocado toast.

Nutritional Information:

- Calories: 380

- Protein: 20g

- Carbohydrates: 25g

- Fiber: 8g

- Sugars: 4g

- Fat: 24g

- Saturated Fat: 5g

- Cholesterol: 370mg

- Sodium: 450mg

2. Greek Yogurt Parfait with Berries and Almonds

Prep Time: 5 minutes

Serving Size: 1

Ingredients:

- 1/2 cup Greek yogurt

- 1/4 cup blueberries

- 1/4 cup strawberries, sliced

- 2 tablespoons almonds, chopped

- 1 tablespoon honey

Instructions:

1. In a glass or bowl, layer Greek yogurt, blueberries, and sliced strawberries.

2. Repeat the layers until the container is filled.

3. Top with chopped almonds and drizzle honey over the parfait.

Nutritional Information:

- Calories: 280

- Protein: 15g

- Carbohydrates: 25g

- Fiber: 4g

- Sugars: 18g

- Fat: 14g

- Saturated Fat: 1g

- Cholesterol: 10mg

- Sodium: 50mg

3. Quinoa Breakfast Bowl with Nuts and Dried Fruits

Prep Time: 15 minutes
Cooking Time: 15 minutes
Serving Size: 1
Ingredients:

- 1/2 cup cooked quinoa

- 1/4 cup mixed nuts (almonds, walnuts)

- 2 tablespoons dried cranberries

- 1/2 banana, sliced

- 1 tablespoon chia seeds

- 1/2 cup almond milk

Instructions:

1. Cook quinoa according to package instructions.

2. In a bowl, combine cooked quinoa, mixed nuts, dried cranberries, banana slices, and chia seeds.

3. Pour almond milk over the mixture and stir well.

4. Allow the mixture to sit for a few minutes to let the chia seeds absorb the liquid.

Nutritional Information:

- Calories: 400

- Protein: 12g

- Carbohydrates: 60g

- Fiber: 10g

- Sugars: 18g

- Fat: 15g

- Saturated Fat: 1g

- Cholesterol: 0mg

- Sodium: 80mg

4. Sweet Potato and Spinach Breakfast Hash

Prep Time: 10 minutes

Cooking Time: 20 minutes

Serving Size: 1

Ingredients:

- 1 small sweet potato, diced

- 1/2 cup spinach, chopped

- 1/4 cup red onion, diced

- 1 clove garlic, minced

- 1 tablespoon olive oil

- 1 egg

- Salt and pepper to taste

Instructions:

1. In a pan, heat olive oil over medium heat.

2. Add sweet potatoes, red onion, and garlic. Cook until sweet potatoes are tender.

3. Add chopped spinach and cook until wilted.

4. Make a well in the center of the pan and crack an egg into it.

5. Cover the pan and cook until the egg is done to your liking.

6. Season with salt and pepper and serve.

Nutritional Information:

- Calories: 380

- Protein: 12g

- Carbohydrates: 35g

- Fiber: 6g

- Sugars: 7g

- Fat: 22g

- Saturated Fat: 4g

- Cholesterol: 210mg

- Sodium: 120mg

5. Whole Grain Pancakes with Fresh Fruit Topping

Prep Time: 15 minutes

Cooking Time: 15 minutes

Serving Size: 2 pancakes

Ingredients:

- 1/2 cup whole wheat flour

- 1/2 cup oat flour

- 1 teaspoon baking powder

- 1/4 teaspoon cinnamon

- 1/2 cup almond milk

- 1 tablespoon maple syrup

- 1 egg

- 1/2 cup mixed berries (blueberries, raspberries)

Instructions:

1. In a bowl, whisk together whole wheat flour, oat flour, baking powder, and cinnamon.

2. In a separate bowl, mix almond milk, maple syrup, and egg.

3. Combine wet and dry ingredients, stirring until just combined.

4. Heat a non-stick pan over medium heat.

5. Pour 1/4 cup of batter onto the pan for each pancake. Cook until bubbles form, then flip and cook the other side.

6. Top pancakes with mixed berries.

Nutritional Information:

- Calories: 350

- Protein: 10g

- Carbohydrates: 60g

- Fiber: 8g

- Sugars: 12g

- Fat: 8g

- Saturated Fat: 1g

- Cholesterol: 50mg

- Sodium: 210mg

6. Spinach and Feta Egg Muffins

Prep Time: 10 minutes

Cooking Time: 20 minutes

Serving Size: 2 muffins

Ingredients:

- 4 large eggs

- 1/2 cup spinach, chopped

- 2 tablespoons feta cheese, crumbled

- 1/4 cup cherry tomatoes, halved

- Salt and pepper to taste

Instructions:

1. Preheat the oven to 350°F (175°C) and grease a muffin tin.

2. In a bowl, whisk eggs and season with salt and pepper.

3. Add chopped spinach, feta cheese, and cherry tomatoes to the eggs. Mix well.

4. Pour the mixture into the muffin tin, filling each cup about halfway.

5. Bake for 15-20 minutes or until the eggs are set.

Nutritional Information:

- Calories: 220

- Protein: 16g

- Carbohydrates: 3g

- Fiber: 1g

- Sugars: 1g

- Fat: 16g

- Saturated Fat: 6g

- Cholesterol: 380mg

- Sodium: 280mg

7. Chia Seed Pudding with Almond Butter and Banana

Prep Time: 5 minutes (plus chilling time)
Serving Size: 1
Ingredients:

- 2 tablespoons chia seeds

- 1/2 cup almond milk

- 1/2 teaspoon vanilla extract

- 1 tablespoon almond butter

- 1/2 banana, sliced

Instructions:

1. In a bowl, mix chia seeds, almond milk, and vanilla extract.

2. Stir well and let it sit for a few minutes, then stir again to prevent clumping.

3. Refrigerate for at least 2 hours or overnight until the mixture thickens.

4. Before serving, top with almond butter and banana slices.

Nutritional Information:

- Calories: 320

- Protein: 10g

- Carbohydrates: 30g

- Fiber: 14g

- Sugars: 8g

- Fat: 18g

- Saturated Fat: 1.5g

- Cholesterol: 0mg

- Sodium: 120mg

8. Cottage Cheese and Pineapple Bowl

Prep Time: 5 minutes

Serving Size: 1

Ingredients:

- 1/2 cup low-fat cottage cheese

- 1/2 cup pineapple chunks (fresh or canned)

- 1 tablespoon flaxseeds

- 1 teaspoon honey

Instructions:

1. In a bowl, combine cottage cheese and pineapple chunks.

2. Sprinkle flaxseeds over the mixture.

3. Drizzle honey on top.

Nutritional Information:

- Calories: 280

- Protein: 20g

- Carbohydrates: 30g

- Fiber: 4g

- Sugars: 24g

- Fat: 10g

- Saturated Fat: 1.5g

- Cholesterol: 10mg

- Sodium: 400mg

9. Avocado and Smoked Salmon Toast

Prep Time: 10 minutes

Serving Size: 1

Ingredients:

- 1 slice whole-grain bread

- 1/2 avocado, mashed

- 2 ounces smoked salmon

- 1 teaspoon capers

- Fresh dill for garnish

- Lemon wedge for serving

Instructions:

1. Toast the whole-grain bread to your liking.

2. Spread mashed avocado on the toasted bread.

3. Top with smoked salmon and sprinkle capers over the salmon.

4. Garnish with fresh dill and serve with a lemon wedge.

Nutritional Information:

- Calories: 320

- Protein: 18g

- Carbohydrates: 20g

- Fiber: 8g

- Sugars: 1g

- Fat: 20g

- Saturated Fat: 3g

- Cholesterol: 15mg

- Sodium: 700mg

10. Mango and Coconut Chia Smoothie

Prep Time: 5 minutes

Serving Size: 1

Ingredients:

- 1/2 cup frozen mango chunks

- 1/2 cup unsweetened coconut milk

- 1/2 cup Greek yogurt

- 2 tablespoons chia seeds

- 1 tablespoon shredded coconut

Instructions:

1. In a blender, combine frozen mango, coconut milk, Greek yogurt, and chia seeds.

2. Blend until smooth.

3. Pour into a glass and sprinkle shredded coconut on top.

Nutritional Information:

- Calories: 350

- Protein: 15g

- Carbohydrates: 40g

- Fiber: 10g

- Sugars: 25g

- Fat: 15g

- Saturated Fat: 8g

- Cholesterol: 10mg

- Sodium: 70mg

11. Egg and Veggie Breakfast Wrap

Prep Time: 10 minutes

Cooking Time: 5 minutes

Serving Size: 1

Ingredients:

- 1 whole-grain tortilla

- 2 large eggs, scrambled

- 1/4 cup black beans, cooked

- 1/4 cup diced bell peppers

- 2 tablespoons salsa

- Fresh cilantro for garnish

Instructions:

1. Heat the tortilla in a dry skillet or microwave until warm.

2. In a pan, scramble the eggs and add black beans and diced bell peppers.

3. Spoon the egg and veggie mixture onto the warm tortilla.

4. Top with salsa and garnish with fresh cilantro.

5. Fold the tortilla to create a wrap.

Nutritional Information:

- Calories: 380

- Protein: 20g

- Carbohydrates: 35g

- Fiber: 8g

- Sugars: 4g

- Fat: 18g

- Saturated Fat: 4.5g

- Cholesterol: 380mg

- Sodium: 480mg

12. Blueberry Almond Chia Pudding

Prep Time: 5 minutes (plus chilling time)

Serving Size: 1

Ingredients:

- 2 tablespoons chia seeds

- 1/2 cup almond milk

- 1/4 teaspoon almond extract

- 1/2 cup blueberries

- 1 tablespoon slivered almonds

Instructions:

1. In a bowl, mix chia seeds, almond milk, and almond extract.

2. Stir well and let it sit for a few minutes, then stir again to prevent clumping.

3. Refrigerate for at least 2 hours or overnight until the mixture thickens.

4. Before serving, top with blueberries and slivered almonds.

Nutritional Information:

- Calories: 300

- Protein: 8g

- Carbohydrates: 30g

- Fiber: 12g

- Sugars: 10g

- Fat: 18g

- Saturated Fat: 1.5g

- Cholesterol: 0mg

- Sodium: 120mg

13. Turkey and Veggie Breakfast Skillet

Prep Time: 10 minutes

Cooking Time: 15 minutes

Serving Size: 1

Ingredients:

- 1/2 cup lean ground turkey

- 1/4 cup diced zucchini

- 1/4 cup diced bell peppers

- 1/4 cup cherry tomatoes, halved

- 1/4 teaspoon cumin

- 1/4 teaspoon paprika

- Salt and pepper to taste

- 1 egg

Instructions:

1. In a skillet, cook ground turkey until browned.

2. Add diced zucchini, bell peppers, and cherry tomatoes to the skillet. Cook until vegetables are tender.

3. Season with cumin, paprika, salt, and pepper.

4. Create a well in the center and crack an egg into it. Cover and cook until the egg is done to your liking.

Nutritional Information:

- Calories: 320

- Protein: 26g

- Carbohydrates: 10g

- Fiber: 3g

- Sugars: 4g

- Fat: 20g

- Saturated Fat: 5g

- Cholesterol: 250mg

- Sodium: 150mg

14. Peanut Butter Banana Overnight Oats

Prep Time: 5 minutes (plus chilling time)

Serving Size: 1

Ingredients:

- 1/2 cup rolled oats

- 1/2 cup almond milk

- 1 tablespoon peanut butter

- 1/2 banana, sliced

- 1 teaspoon chia seeds

Instructions:

1. In a jar, combine rolled oats, almond milk, peanut butter, banana slices, and chia seeds.

2. Stir well, cover, and refrigerate overnight.

3. In the morning, give the oats a good stir and enjoy.

Nutritional Information:

- Calories: 380

- Protein: 13g

- Carbohydrates: 50g

- Fiber: 10g

- Sugars: 10g

- Fat: 15g

- Saturated Fat: 2g

- Cholesterol: 0mg

- Sodium: 180mg

15. Tomato and Basil Frittata

Prep Time: 10 minutes

Cooking Time: 20 minutes

Serving Size: 2

Ingredients:

- 4 large eggs

- 1/2 cup cherry tomatoes, halved

- 2 tablespoons fresh basil, chopped

- 1/4 cup feta cheese, crumbled

- Salt and pepper to taste

Instructions:

1. Preheat the oven to 350°F (175°C).

2. In a bowl, whisk eggs and season with salt and pepper.

3. Add cherry tomatoes, fresh basil, and feta cheese to the eggs. Mix well.

4. Pour the mixture into a greased oven-safe skillet.

5. Bake for 15-20 minutes or until the frittata is set.

Nutritional Information:

- Calories: 280

- Protein: 18g

- Carbohydrates: 5g

- Fiber: 1g

- Sugars: 2g

- Fat: 20g

- Saturated Fat: 7g

- Cholesterol: 380mg

- Sodium: 300mg

16. Cinnamon Apple Walnut Porridge

Prep Time: 10 minutes

Cooking Time: 10 minutes

Serving Size: 1

Ingredients:

- 1/2 cup old-fashioned oats

- 1/2 cup unsweetened almond milk

- 1/2 apple, diced

- 1/4 teaspoon cinnamon

- 1 tablespoon chopped walnuts

- 1 teaspoon maple syrup

Instructions:

1. In a saucepan, combine oats, almond milk, diced apple, and cinnamon.

2. Cook over medium heat until the oats are tender.

3. Stir in chopped walnuts and drizzle with maple syrup before serving.

Nutritional Information:

- Calories: 320

- Protein: 9g

- Carbohydrates: 50g

- Fiber: 8g

- Sugars: 16g

- Fat: 11g

- Saturated Fat: 1g

- Cholesterol: 0mg

- Sodium: 80mg

17. Mushroom and Spinach Breakfast Wrap

Prep Time: 10 minutes

Cooking Time: 10 minutes

Serving Size: 1

Ingredients:

- 1 whole-grain tortilla

- 1/2 cup sliced mushrooms

- 1 cup fresh spinach

- 1/4 cup red bell pepper, sliced

- 1 tablespoon feta cheese, crumbled

- 1 teaspoon olive oil

Instructions:

1. In a pan, sauté mushrooms, spinach, and red bell pepper in olive oil until tender.

2. Warm the whole-grain tortilla.

3. Spoon the sautéed vegetables onto the tortilla.

4. Sprinkle crumbled feta cheese on top.

5. Fold the tortilla to create a wrap.

Nutritional Information:

- Calories: 280

- Protein: 12g

- Carbohydrates: 35g

- Fiber: 8g

- Sugars: 5g

- Fat: 12g

- Saturated Fat: 3g

- Cholesterol: 15mg

- Sodium: 350mg

18. Protein-Packed Breakfast Burrito

Prep Time: 15 minutes

Cooking Time: 10 minutes

Serving Size: 1

Ingredients:

- 1 whole-grain tortilla

- 1/2 cup black beans, cooked

- 2 large eggs, scrambled

- 1/4 cup diced tomatoes

- 2 tablespoons shredded cheddar cheese

- Salsa for topping

Instructions:

1. Heat the whole-grain tortilla in a dry skillet or microwave until warm.

2. In a pan, scramble the eggs and cook until done.

3. Assemble the burrito by placing black beans, scrambled eggs, diced tomatoes, and shredded cheddar cheese on the tortilla.

4. Top with salsa before folding into a burrito.

Nutritional Information:

- Calories: 420

- Protein: 24g

- Carbohydrates: 45g

- Fiber: 10g

- Sugars: 5g

- Fat: 18g

- Saturated Fat: 7g

- Cholesterol: 380mg

- Sodium: 550mg

19. Salmon and Cream Cheese Bagel

Prep Time: 10 minutes

Cooking Time: 5 minutes

Serving Size: 1

Ingredients:

- 1 whole grain bagel, sliced and toasted

- 2 ounces smoked salmon

- 2 tablespoons cream cheese

- 1 tablespoon capers

- Fresh dill for garnish

Instructions:

1. Toast the whole grain bagel until golden brown.

2. Spread cream cheese on each half of the bagel.

3. Place smoked salmon on top of the cream cheese.

4. Sprinkle capers over the salmon and garnish with fresh dill.

Nutritional Information:

- Calories: 350

- Protein: 20g

- Carbohydrates: 40g

- Fiber: 6g

- Sugars: 5g

- Fat: 14g

- Saturated Fat: 7g

- Cholesterol: 30mg

- Sodium: 700mg

20. Coconut Berry Breakfast Bowl

Prep Time: 10 minutes

Serving Size: 1

Ingredients:

- 1/2 cup cooked quinoa

- 1/2 cup coconut milk

- 1/2 cup mixed berries (strawberries, blueberries, raspberries)

- 1 tablespoon shredded coconut

- 1 tablespoon chopped almonds

Instructions:

1. In a bowl, combine cooked quinoa and coconut milk.

2. Top with mixed berries, shredded coconut, and chopped almonds.

Nutritional Information:

- Calories: 300

- Protein: 8g

- Carbohydrates: 35g

- Fiber: 6g

- Sugars: 6g

- Fat: 15g

- Saturated Fat: 8g

- Cholesterol: 0mg

- Sodium: 10mg

CHAPTER 5: LUNCH RECIPES

1. Grilled Chicken Salad with Citrus Vinaigrette

Prep Time: 15 minutes

Cooking Time: 15 minutes

Serving Size: 1

Ingredients:

- 4 ounces grilled chicken breast, sliced

- 2 cups mixed salad greens

- 1/2 cup cherry tomatoes, halved

- 1/4 cup cucumber, sliced

- 1/4 cup red bell pepper, sliced

- 1/4 cup feta cheese, crumbled

- 2 tablespoons olive oil

- 1 tablespoon orange juice

- 1 teaspoon Dijon mustard

- Salt and pepper to taste

Instructions:

1. In a large bowl, combine salad greens, cherry tomatoes, cucumber, red bell pepper, and grilled chicken.

2. In a small bowl, whisk together olive oil, orange juice, Dijon mustard, salt, and pepper to create the vinaigrette.

3. Drizzle the vinaigrette over the salad and toss gently.

4. Top with crumbled feta cheese before serving.

Nutritional Information:

- Calories: 450

- Protein: 30g

- Carbohydrates: 15g

- Fiber: 5g

- Sugars: 8g

- Fat: 30g

- Saturated Fat: 7g

- Cholesterol: 80mg

- Sodium: 400mg

2. Salmon and Quinoa Bowl with Roasted Vegetables

Prep Time: 20 minutes

Cooking Time: 25 minutes

Serving Size: 1

Ingredients:

- 4 ounces salmon fillet

- 1/2 cup quinoa, cooked

- 1 cup mixed vegetables (zucchini, cherry tomatoes, bell peppers)

- 1 tablespoon olive oil

- 1 teaspoon lemon juice

- 1/2 teaspoon dried dill

- Salt and pepper to taste

Instructions:

1. Preheat the oven to 400°F (200°C).

2. Place salmon fillet on a baking sheet, surrounded by mixed vegetables.

3. Drizzle olive oil and lemon juice over the salmon and vegetables. Sprinkle with dried dill, salt, and pepper.

4. Roast in the oven for 20-25 minutes or until salmon is cooked through.

5. Serve over a bed of cooked quinoa.

Nutritional Information:

- Calories: 480

- Protein: 30g

- Carbohydrates: 40g

- Fiber: 6g

- Sugars: 5g

- Fat: 22g

- Saturated Fat: 4g

- Cholesterol: 70mg

- Sodium: 120mg

3. Turkey and Vegetable Stir-Fry with Brown Rice

Prep Time: 15 minutes

Cooking Time: 15 minutes

Serving Size: 1

Ingredients:

- 1/2 cup lean ground turkey

- 1 cup mixed stir-fry vegetables (broccoli, carrots, snow peas)

- 1 cup cooked brown rice

- 1 tablespoon soy sauce (low sodium)

- 1 teaspoon sesame oil

- 1/2 teaspoon ginger, minced

- 1 clove garlic, minced

Instructions:

1. In a wok or large skillet, cook ground turkey until browned.

2. Add mixed vegetables, ginger, and garlic. Stir-fry until vegetables are tender-crisp.

3. Add cooked brown rice to the wok and stir.

4. Drizzle soy sauce and sesame oil over the mixture. Continue stirring until well combined.

Nutritional Information:

- Calories: 420

- Protein: 25g

- Carbohydrates: 55g

- Fiber: 8g

- Sugars: 3g

- Fat: 12g

- Saturated Fat: 2g

- Cholesterol: 50mg

- Sodium: 600mg

4. Mediterranean Chickpea Salad

Prep Time: 15 minutes

Serving Size: 1

Ingredients:

- 1 cup canned chickpeas, drained and rinsed

- 1/2 cucumber, diced

- 1/2 cup cherry tomatoes, halved

- 1/4 cup red onion, finely chopped

- 1/4 cup Kalamata olives, sliced

- 2 tablespoons feta cheese, crumbled

- 1 tablespoon olive oil

- 1 tablespoon balsamic vinegar

- 1 teaspoon dried oregano

- Salt and pepper to taste

Instructions:

1. In a large bowl, combine chickpeas, cucumber, cherry tomatoes, red onion, olives, and feta cheese.

2. In a small bowl, whisk together olive oil, balsamic vinegar, dried oregano, salt, and pepper.

3. Pour the dressing over the salad and toss gently before serving.

Nutritional Information:

- Calories: 380

- Protein: 15g

- Carbohydrates: 45g

- Fiber: 12g

- Sugars: 8g

- Fat: 18g

- Saturated Fat: 4g

- Cholesterol: 15mg

- Sodium: 500mg

5. Vegetarian Quinoa and Black Bean Stuffed Peppers

Prep Time: 20 minutes
Cooking Time: 30 minutes
Serving Size: 1
Ingredients:

- 2 large bell peppers, halved and seeds removed

- 1/2 cup quinoa, cooked

- 1/2 cup black beans, cooked

- 1/4 cup corn kernels

- 1/4 cup diced tomatoes

- 1/4 cup red onion, finely chopped

- 1/2 teaspoon cumin

- 1/2 teaspoon chili powder

- Salt and pepper to taste

- 2 tablespoons shredded cheddar cheese

Instructions:

1. Preheat the oven to 375°F (190°C).

2. In a bowl, combine cooked quinoa, black beans, corn, tomatoes, red onion, cumin, chili powder, salt, and pepper.

3. Stuff each bell pepper half with the quinoa and black bean mixture.

4. Sprinkle shredded cheddar cheese on top.

5. Bake for 25-30 minutes or until the peppers are tender.

Nutritional Information:

- Calories: 420

- Protein: 20g

- Carbohydrates: 65g

- Fiber: 12g

- Sugars: 6g

- Fat: 10g

- Saturated Fat: 3.5g

- Cholesterol: 15mg

- Sodium: 400mg

6. Shrimp and Broccoli Stir-Fry with Cauliflower Rice

Prep Time: 15 minutes

Cooking Time: 15 minutes

Serving Size: 1

Ingredients:

- 6 ounces shrimp, peeled and deveined

- 1 cup broccoli florets

- 1 cup cauliflower rice

- 1/2 cup bell peppers, sliced

- 1 tablespoon low-sodium soy sauce

- 1 tablespoon hoisin sauce

- 1 teaspoon sesame oil

- 1/2 teaspoon garlic, minced

- 1/2 teaspoon ginger, minced

- Green onions for garnish

Instructions:

1. In a wok or skillet, stir-fry shrimp until cooked through. Set aside.

2. Stir-fry broccoli, cauliflower rice, and bell peppers until vegetables are tender-crisp.

3. Add cooked shrimp back to the wok.

4. In a small bowl, mix soy sauce, hoisin sauce, sesame oil, garlic, and ginger. Pour over the shrimp and vegetables. Toss until well coated.

5. Garnish with chopped green onions before serving.

Nutritional Information:

- Calories: 380

- Protein: 30g

- Carbohydrates: 35g

- Fiber: 10g

- Sugars: 10g

- Fat: 15g

- Saturated Fat: 2g

- Cholesterol: 200mg

- Sodium: 700mg

7. Lentil and Vegetable Soup

Prep Time: 20 minutes

Cooking Time: 30 minutes

Serving Size: 1

Ingredients:

- 1/2 cup lentils, rinsed and drained

- 1/2 cup carrots, diced

- 1/2 cup celery, diced

- 1/2 cup onion, finely chopped

- 2 cloves garlic, minced

- 4 cups low-sodium vegetable broth

- 1 cup spinach, chopped

- 1 teaspoon cumin

- 1/2 teaspoon turmeric

- Salt and pepper to taste

Instructions:

1. In a large pot, sauté onions and garlic until softened.

2. Add lentils, carrots, celery, cumin, turmeric, salt, and pepper. Stir to combine.

3. Pour in vegetable broth and bring to a boil. Reduce heat and simmer for 25-30 minutes or until lentils are tender.

4. Add chopped spinach and cook until wilted before serving.

Nutritional Information:

- Calories: 320

- Protein: 18g

- Carbohydrates: 55g

- Fiber: 18g

- Sugars: 7g

- Fat: 2g

- Saturated Fat: 0g

- Cholesterol: 0mg

- Sodium: 500mg

8. Caprese Chicken Skewers

Prep Time: 15 minutes

Cooking Time: 10 minutes

Serving Size: 1

Ingredients:

- 4 ounces chicken breast, cut into cubes

- 1 cup cherry tomatoes

- 1/2 cup fresh mozzarella balls

- Fresh basil leaves

- 1 tablespoon balsamic glaze

- 1 tablespoon olive oil

- Salt and pepper to taste

Instructions:

1. Thread chicken, cherry tomatoes, and mozzarella balls onto skewers.

2. Drizzle olive oil over the skewers and season with salt and pepper.

3. Grill or broil for 8-10 minutes or until chicken is cooked through.

4. Arrange the skewers on a plate, garnish with fresh basil, and drizzle balsamic glaze before serving.

Nutritional Information:

- Calories: 380

- Protein: 30g

- Carbohydrates: 8g

- Fiber: 2g

- Sugars: 5g

- Fat: 25g

- Saturated Fat: 8g

- Cholesterol: 80mg

- Sodium: 350mg

9. Eggplant and Tomato Stew with Quinoa

Prep Time: 20 minutes

Cooking Time: 30 minutes

Serving Size: 1

Ingredients:

- 1 small eggplant, diced

- 1 cup cherry tomatoes, halved

- 1/2 cup quinoa, cooked

- 1/4 cup red onion, finely chopped

- 2 cloves garlic, minced

- 1/2 cup vegetable broth

- 1 teaspoon dried oregano

- 1/2 teaspoon red pepper flakes

- Salt and pepper to taste

- Fresh parsley for garnish

Instructions:

1. In a pot, sauté red onion and garlic until softened.

2. Add diced eggplant, cherry tomatoes, oregano, red pepper flakes, salt, and pepper. Cook for 5 minutes.

3. Pour in vegetable broth and simmer until eggplant is tender.

4. Serve the stew over a bed of cooked quinoa and garnish with fresh parsley.

Nutritional Information:

- Calories: 340

- Protein: 12g

- Carbohydrates: 55g

- Fiber: 10g

- Sugars: 8g

- Fat: 10g

- Saturated Fat: 1g

- Cholesterol: 0mg

- Sodium: 250mg

10. Chicken and Vegetable Wrap with Hummus

Prep Time: 15 minutes

Cooking Time: 10 minutes

Serving Size: 1

Ingredients:

- 4 ounces grilled chicken breast, sliced

- 1 whole-grain wrap

- 1/2 cup mixed salad greens

- 1/4 cup cucumber, sliced

- 1/4 cup cherry tomatoes, halved

- 2 tablespoons hummus

- 1 tablespoon feta cheese, crumbled

Instructions:

1. Lay the whole-grain wrap on a flat surface.

2. Spread hummus evenly over the wrap.

3. Layer with mixed salad greens, sliced grilled chicken, cucumber, cherry tomatoes, and crumbled feta cheese.

4. Fold the sides of the wrap and roll tightly.

Nutritional Information:

- Calories: 420

- Protein: 30g

- Carbohydrates: 40g

- Fiber: 8g

- Sugars: 6g

- Fat: 18g

- Saturated Fat: 4g

- Cholesterol: 80mg

- Sodium: 600mg

11. Vegetable and Tofu Stir-Fry with Brown Rice

Prep Time: 20 minutes

Cooking Time: 15 minutes

Serving Size: 1

Ingredients:

- 1/2 cup extra-firm tofu, cubed

- 1 cup mixed stir-fry vegetables (broccoli, carrots, snap peas)

- 1 cup cooked brown rice

- 1 tablespoon low-sodium soy sauce

71

- 1 tablespoon hoisin sauce

- 1 teaspoon sesame oil

- 1/2 teaspoon garlic, minced

- 1/2 teaspoon ginger, minced

Instructions:

1. Press tofu to remove excess water and cut into cubes.

2. In a wok or skillet, stir-fry tofu until golden brown. Set aside.

3. Stir-fry mixed vegetables until tender-crisp.

4. Add cooked brown rice and tofu to the wok.

5. In a small bowl, mix soy sauce, hoisin sauce, sesame oil, garlic, and ginger. Pour over the mixture and toss until well combined.

Nutritional Information:

- Calories: 400

- Protein: 18g

- Carbohydrates: 55g

- Fiber: 8g

- Sugars: 3g

- Fat: 12g

- Saturated Fat: 2g

- Cholesterol: 0mg

- Sodium: 600mg

12. Greek Turkey Burger with Sweet Potato Wedges

Prep Time: 20 minutes

Cooking Time: 25 minutes

Serving Size: 1

Ingredients:

- 4 ounces lean ground turkey

- 1 whole-grain burger bun

- 1/4 cup cucumber, sliced

- 1/4 cup cherry tomatoes, halved

- 2 tablespoons feta cheese, crumbled

- 1 tablespoon Greek yogurt

- 1 sweet potato, cut into wedges

- 1 tablespoon olive oil

- 1/2 teaspoon dried oregano

- Salt and pepper to taste

Instructions:

1. Preheat the oven to 400°F (200°C).

2. Toss sweet potato wedges with olive oil, dried oregano, salt, and pepper. Roast for 20-25 minutes or until golden brown.

3. Season ground turkey with salt and pepper, then shape into a patty.

4. Grill or pan-fry the turkey burger until fully cooked.

5. Assemble the burger with cucumber slices, cherry tomatoes, feta cheese, and a dollop of Greek yogurt. Serve with sweet potato wedges.

Nutritional Information:

- Calories: 480
- Protein: 25g
- Carbohydrates: 55g
- Fiber: 8g
- Sugars: 8g
- Fat: 18g
- Saturated Fat: 5g
- Cholesterol: 60mg
- Sodium: 550mg

13. Sesame Ginger Salmon with Broccoli and Quinoa

Prep Time: 20 minutes

Cooking Time: 20 minutes

Serving Size: 1

Ingredients:

- 4 ounces salmon fillet

- 1/2 cup quinoa, cooked

- 1 cup broccoli florets

- 1 tablespoon low-sodium soy sauce

- 1 tablespoon rice vinegar

- 1 teaspoon sesame oil

- 1/2 teaspoon ginger, minced

- 1 clove garlic, minced

- Sesame seeds for garnish

Instructions:

1. Preheat the oven to 400°F (200°C).

2. Place salmon fillet on a baking sheet and surround with broccoli florets.

3. In a small bowl, whisk together soy sauce, rice vinegar, sesame oil, ginger, and garlic.

4. Brush the salmon with the sauce and drizzle the remaining sauce over the broccoli.

5. Bake for 15-20 minutes or until salmon is cooked through.

6. Serve over a bed of cooked quinoa and garnish with sesame seeds.

Nutritional Information:

- Calories: 450

- Protein: 30g

- Carbohydrates: 40g

- Fiber: 6g

- Sugars: 3g

- Fat: 20g

- Saturated Fat: 3.5g

- Cholesterol: 80mg

- Sodium: 500mg

14. Chickpea and Spinach Curry with Brown Rice

Prep Time: 20 minutes

Cooking Time: 25 minutes

Serving Size: 1

Ingredients:

- 1/2 cup canned chickpeas, drained and rinsed

- 1 cup spinach leaves

- 1/2 cup tomatoes, diced

- 1/4 cup red onion, finely chopped

- 1/2 cup light coconut milk

- 1 tablespoon curry powder

- 1/2 teaspoon turmeric

- 1/2 teaspoon cumin

- Salt and pepper to taste

- 1 cup cooked brown rice

Instructions:

1. In a pan, sauté red onion until softened.

2. Add chickpeas, tomatoes, curry powder, turmeric, cumin, salt, and pepper. Cook for 5 minutes.

3. Pour in light coconut milk and bring to a simmer.

4. Stir in spinach leaves and cook until wilted.

5. Serve the curry over a bed of cooked brown rice.

Nutritional Information:

- Calories: 400

- Protein: 15g

- Carbohydrates: 60g

- Fiber: 12g

- Sugars: 6g

- Fat: 10g

- Saturated Fat: 5g

- Cholesterol: 0mg

- Sodium: 500mg

15. Pesto Chicken and Vegetable Skewers with Quinoa

Prep Time: 15 minutes

Cooking Time: 15 minutes

Serving Size: 1

Ingredients:

- 4 ounces chicken breast, cut into cubes

- 1/2 cup cherry tomatoes

- 1/2 cup zucchini, sliced

- 1/4 cup red onion, sliced

- 2 tablespoons pesto sauce

- 1 tablespoon olive oil

- 1 cup quinoa, cooked

- Fresh basil leaves for garnish

Instructions:

1. Thread chicken, cherry tomatoes, zucchini, and red onion onto skewers.

2. In a small bowl, mix pesto sauce and olive oil.

3. Brush the skewers with the pesto mixture.

4. Grill or broil for 10-15 minutes or until chicken is cooked through.

5. Serve over a bed of cooked quinoa and garnish with fresh basil leaves.

Nutritional Information:

- Calories: 450

- Protein: 30g

- Carbohydrates: 40g

- Fiber: 6g

- Sugars: 3g

- Fat: 20g

- Saturated Fat: 3.5g

- Cholesterol: 80mg

- Sodium: 350mg

16. Mushroom and Spinach Stuffed Chicken Breast with Sweet Potato Mash

Prep Time: 25 minutes

Cooking Time: 30 minutes

Serving Size: 1

Ingredients:

- 6 ounces chicken breast

- 1/2 cup mushrooms, chopped

- 1 cup spinach, chopped

- 1 clove garlic, minced

- 1/4 cup mozzarella cheese, shredded

- 1 sweet potato, peeled and diced

- 1 tablespoon butter

- 1 tablespoon almond milk

- Salt and pepper to taste

- Fresh parsley for garnish

Instructions:

1. Preheat the oven to 375°F (190°C).

2. In a skillet, sauté mushrooms, spinach, and garlic until wilted. Set aside.

3. Cut a pocket into the side of the chicken breast and stuff with the mushroom and spinach mixture. Secure with toothpicks if needed.

4. Season the chicken with salt and pepper and place in a baking dish.

5. Bake for 25-30 minutes or until the chicken is cooked through.

6. Meanwhile, boil sweet potatoes until tender. Mash with butter, almond milk, salt, and pepper.

7. Serve the stuffed chicken breast over a bed of sweet potato mash, garnished with fresh parsley.

Nutritional Information:

- Calories: 480

- Protein: 35g

- Carbohydrates: 40g

- Fiber: 8g

- Sugars: 8g

- Fat: 20g

- Saturated Fat: 8g

- Cholesterol: 100mg

- Sodium: 350mg

17. Teriyaki Tofu and Vegetable Skewers with Brown Rice

Prep Time: 20 minutes

Cooking Time: 15 minutes

Serving Size: 1

Ingredients:

- 1/2 cup extra-firm tofu, cubed

- 1 cup mixed vegetables (bell peppers, zucchini, mushrooms)

- 1/2 cup pineapple chunks

- 1/4 cup teriyaki sauce (low sodium)

- 1 cup cooked brown rice

- Sesame seeds for garnish

Instructions:

1. In a bowl, marinate tofu, mixed vegetables, and pineapple chunks in teriyaki sauce.

2. Thread tofu, vegetables, and pineapple onto skewers.

3. Grill or broil for 10-15 minutes, turning occasionally, until vegetables are tender.

4. Serve over a bed of cooked brown rice and sprinkle with sesame seeds.

Nutritional Information:

- Calories: 420

- Protein: 15g

- Carbohydrates: 65g

- Fiber: 8g

- Sugars: 12g

- Fat: 10g

- Saturated Fat: 1.5g

- Cholesterol: 0mg

- Sodium: 600mg

18. Quinoa and Black Bean Bowl with Avocado Salsa

Prep Time: 15 minutes

Cooking Time: 15 minutes

Serving Size: 1

Ingredients:

- 1/2 cup quinoa, cooked

- 1/2 cup black beans, cooked

- 1/4 cup corn kernels

- 1/4 cup red bell pepper, diced

- 1/4 cup cherry tomatoes, halved

- 1/2 avocado, diced

- 1 tablespoon cilantro, chopped

- 1 tablespoon lime juice

- Salt and pepper to taste

Instructions:

1. In a bowl, combine quinoa, black beans, corn, red bell pepper, and cherry tomatoes.

2. In a separate bowl, mix diced avocado, cilantro, lime juice, salt, and pepper to create the salsa.

3. Spoon the quinoa and black bean mixture into a bowl and top with avocado salsa.

Nutritional Information:

- Calories: 380

- Protein: 15g

- Carbohydrates: 55g

- Fiber: 12g

- Sugars: 5g

- Fat: 15g

- Saturated Fat: 2g

- Cholesterol: 0mg

- Sodium: 300mg

19. Vegetarian Fajita Bowl with Cauliflower Rice

Prep Time: 20 minutes

Cooking Time: 15 minutes

Serving Size: 1

Ingredients:

- 1/2 cup cauliflower rice, cooked

- 1/2 cup black beans, cooked

- 1/4 cup bell peppers, sliced

- 1/4 cup red onion, sliced

- 1/2 cup cherry tomatoes, halved

- 1/4 cup corn kernels

- 1/2 avocado, sliced

- 1 tablespoon olive oil

- 1 teaspoon taco seasoning

- Fresh cilantro for garnish

Instructions:

1. In a skillet, sauté bell peppers, red onion, cherry tomatoes, and corn in olive oil until tender.

2. Stir in black beans and taco seasoning, cooking for an additional 3-5 minutes.

3. Serve the fajita mixture over a bed of cooked cauliflower rice.

4. Top with sliced avocado and garnish with fresh cilantro.

Nutritional Information:

- Calories: 400

- Protein: 15g

- Carbohydrates: 60g

- Fiber: 15g

- Sugars: 8g

- Fat: 15g

- Saturated Fat: 2g

- Cholesterol: 0mg

- Sodium: 350mg

20. Mango Chicken Lettuce Wraps

Prep Time: 20 minutes

Cooking Time: 15 minutes

Serving Size: 1

Ingredients:

- 4 ounces chicken breast, cooked and shredded

- 1/2 mango, diced

- 1/4 cup red bell pepper, diced

- 2 tablespoons red onion, finely chopped

- 1 tablespoon cilantro, chopped

- 1 tablespoon lime juice

- Lettuce leaves for wrapping

Instructions:

1. In a bowl, combine shredded chicken, diced mango, red bell pepper, red onion, cilantro, and lime juice.

2. Mix until well combined.

3. Spoon the mixture onto lettuce leaves to create wraps.

Nutritional Information:

- Calories: 380

- Protein: 30g

- Carbohydrates: 40g

- Fiber: 6g

- Sugars: 18g

- Fat: 12g

- Saturated Fat: 2.5g

- Cholesterol: 80mg

- Sodium: 350mg

CHAPTER 6: DINNER RECIPES

1. Baked Herb-Crusted Salmon with Roasted Vegetables

Prep Time: 15 minutes
Cooking Time: 20 minutes
Serving Size: 1
Ingredients:

- 6 ounces salmon fillet

- 1 cup mixed vegetables (zucchini, cherry tomatoes, bell peppers)

- 1 tablespoon olive oil

- 1 teaspoon dried herbs (rosemary, thyme, oregano)

- Salt and pepper to taste

Instructions:

1. Preheat the oven to 400°F (200°C).

2. Place salmon fillet on a baking sheet surrounded by mixed vegetables.

3. Drizzle olive oil over the salmon and vegetables. Sprinkle dried herbs, salt, and pepper.

4. Bake for 20 minutes or until salmon is cooked through.

Nutritional Information:

- Calories: 450

- Protein: 30g

- Carbohydrates: 15g

- Fiber: 6g

- Sugars: 5g

- Fat: 30g

- Saturated Fat: 5g

- Cholesterol: 80mg

- Sodium: 400mg

2. Turkey and Vegetable Skillet Stir-Fry

Prep Time: 15 minutes
Cooking Time: 15 minutes
Serving Size: 1
Ingredients:

- 1/2 cup lean ground turkey

- 1 cup mixed stir-fry vegetables (broccoli, carrots, snap peas)

- 1 tablespoon low-sodium soy sauce

- 1 teaspoon sesame oil

- 1/2 teaspoon ginger, minced

- 1/2 teaspoon garlic, minced

- 1 cup cooked brown rice

Instructions:

1. In a skillet, cook ground turkey until browned.

2. Add mixed vegetables, ginger, and garlic. Stir-fry until vegetables are tender-crisp.

3. Drizzle soy sauce and sesame oil over the mixture.

4. Add cooked brown rice and stir until well combined.

Nutritional Information:

- Calories: 420

- Protein: 25g

- Carbohydrates: 55g

- Fiber: 8g

- Sugars: 3g

- Fat: 12g

- Saturated Fat: 2g

- Cholesterol: 50mg

- Sodium: 600mg

3. Spinach and Feta Stuffed Chicken Breast

Prep Time: 20 minutes
Cooking Time: 25 minutes
Serving Size: 1
Ingredients:

- 6 ounces chicken breast

- 1 cup fresh spinach, chopped

- 2 tablespoons feta cheese, crumbled

- 1 clove garlic, minced

- 1/2 teaspoon dried oregano

- Salt and pepper to taste

- 1 teaspoon olive oil

Instructions:

1. Preheat the oven to 375°F (190°C).

2. In a bowl, mix chopped spinach, feta cheese, minced garlic, dried oregano, salt, and pepper.

3. Cut a pocket into the side of the chicken breast and stuff with the spinach and feta mixture.

4. Brush the chicken breast with olive oil and bake for 25 minutes or until cooked through.

Nutritional Information:

- Calories: 380

- Protein: 35g

- Carbohydrates: 5g

- Fiber: 2g

- Sugars: 1g

- Fat: 22g

- Saturated Fat: 7g

- Cholesterol: 100mg

- Sodium: 400mg

4. Vegetarian Lentil Soup

Prep Time: 20 minutes
Cooking Time: 30 minutes
Serving Size: 1
Ingredients:

- 1/2 cup lentils, rinsed and drained

- 1/2 cup carrots, diced

- 1/2 cup celery, diced

- 1/2 cup onion, finely chopped

- 2 cloves garlic, minced

- 4 cups low-sodium vegetable broth

- 1 cup spinach, chopped

- 1 teaspoon cumin

- 1/2 teaspoon turmeric

- Salt and pepper to taste

Instructions:

1. In a large pot, sauté onions and garlic until softened.

2. Add lentils, carrots, celery, cumin, turmeric, salt, and pepper. Stir to combine.

3. Pour in vegetable broth and bring to a boil. Reduce heat and simmer for 25-30 minutes or until lentils are tender.

4. Add chopped spinach and cook until wilted before serving.

Nutritional Information:

- Calories: 320

- Protein: 18g

- Carbohydrates: 55g

- Fiber: 18g

- Sugars: 7g

- Fat: 2g

- Saturated Fat: 0g

- Cholesterol: 0mg

- Sodium: 500mg

5. Mushroom and Spinach Quinoa Risotto

Prep Time: 20 minutes
Cooking Time: 30 minutes
Serving Size: 1
Ingredients:

- 1/2 cup quinoa, uncooked

- 1 cup mushrooms, sliced

- 1 cup fresh spinach

- 1/4 cup Parmesan cheese, grated

- 1/2 cup low-sodium vegetable broth

- 1/2 cup white wine (optional)

- 1 clove garlic, minced

- 1 tablespoon olive oil

- Salt and pepper to taste

Instructions:

1. Rinse quinoa under cold water. Set aside.

2. In a pan, sauté mushrooms and garlic in olive oil until mushrooms are tender.

3. Add quinoa to the pan and toast for 2-3 minutes.

4. Pour in white wine (if using) and cook until mostly evaporated.

5. Gradually add vegetable broth, stirring continuously until quinoa is cooked.

6. Fold in fresh spinach and Parmesan cheese. Season with salt and pepper before serving.

Nutritional Information:

- Calories: 380

- Protein: 15g

- Carbohydrates: 55g

- Fiber: 8g

- Sugars: 3g

- Fat: 12g

- Saturated Fat: 3g

- Cholesterol: 10mg

- Sodium: 400mg

6. Grilled Vegetable and Chicken Skewers with Quinoa

Prep Time: 25 minutes
Cooking Time: 15 minutes
Serving Size: 1
Ingredients:

- 4 ounces chicken breast, cut into cubes

- 1/2 cup zucchini, sliced

- 1/2 cup cherry tomatoes

- 1/4 cup red onion, sliced

- 1/4 cup bell peppers, sliced

- 1 cup quinoa, cooked

- 1 tablespoon olive oil

- 1 teaspoon dried Italian herbs

- Salt and pepper to taste

Instructions:

1. Thread chicken, zucchini, cherry tomatoes, red onion, and bell peppers onto skewers.

2. Drizzle olive oil over the skewers and sprinkle dried Italian herbs, salt, and pepper.

3. Grill for 10-15 minutes or until chicken is cooked through.

4. Serve over a bed of cooked quinoa.

Nutritional Information:

- Calories: 420

- Protein: 30g

- Carbohydrates: 40g

- Fiber: 6g

- Sugars: 5g

- Fat: 18g

- Saturated Fat: 3g

- Cholesterol: 80mg

- Sodium: 350mg

7. Shrimp and Asparagus Stir-Fry with Brown Rice

Prep Time: 15 minutes
Cooking Time: 15 minutes
Serving Size: 1
Ingredients:

- 4 ounces shrimp, peeled and deveined

- 1 cup asparagus, cut into pieces

- 1/2 cup bell peppers, sliced
- 1 cup cooked brown rice
- 1 tablespoon low-sodium soy sauce
- 1 tablespoon oyster sauce
- 1/2 teaspoon ginger, minced
- 1/2 teaspoon garlic, minced
- 1 tablespoon olive oil

Instructions:

1. In a wok or skillet, stir-fry shrimp until cooked through. Set aside.
2. Stir-fry asparagus and bell peppers in olive oil until tender-crisp.
3. Add cooked shrimp back to the wok.
4. In a small bowl, mix soy sauce, oyster sauce, ginger, and garlic. Pour over the shrimp and vegetables. Toss until well coated.
5. Serve over a bed of cooked brown rice.

Nutritional Information:

- Calories: 380
- Protein: 30g
- Carbohydrates: 45g
- Fiber: 8g
- Sugars: 4g
- Fat: 12g
- Saturated Fat: 2g

- Cholesterol: 200mg

- Sodium: 700mg

8. Sweet Potato and Black Bean Chili

Prep Time: 20 minutes
Cooking Time: 30 minutes
Serving Size: 1
Ingredients:

- 1/2 cup black beans, cooked

- 1/2 cup sweet potatoes, diced

- 1/4 cup red bell pepper, diced

- 1/4 cup onion, finely chopped

- 1/2 cup diced tomatoes

- 1 clove garlic, minced

- 1 cup low-sodium vegetable broth

- 1 tablespoon chili powder

- 1/2 teaspoon cumin

- Salt and pepper to taste

Instructions:

1. In a pot, sauté onions and garlic until softened.

2. Add sweet potatoes, red bell pepper, diced tomatoes, chili powder, cumin, salt, and pepper. Cook for 5 minutes.

3. Pour in vegetable broth and simmer until sweet potatoes are tender.

4. Stir in cooked black beans before serving.

Nutritional Information:

- Calories: 360

- Protein: 15g

- Carbohydrates: 65g

- Fiber: 15g

- Sugars: 8g

- Fat: 5g

- Saturated Fat: 1g

- Cholesterol: 0mg

- Sodium: 400mg

9. Cauliflower and Chickpea Curry with Brown Rice

Prep Time: 20 minutes
Cooking Time: 25 minutes
Serving Size: 1
Ingredients:

- 1/2 cup cauliflower florets

- 1/2 cup canned chickpeas, drained and rinsed

- 1/2 cup cherry tomatoes, halved

- 1/4 cup red onion, finely chopped

- 1/2 cup light coconut milk

- 1 tablespoon curry powder

- 1/2 teaspoon turmeric

- 1/2 teaspoon cumin

- Salt and pepper to taste

- 1 cup cooked brown rice

Instructions:

1. In a pan, sauté red onion until softened.
2. Add cauliflower florets, chickpeas, cherry tomatoes, curry powder, turmeric, cumin, salt, and pepper. Cook for 5 minutes.
3. Pour in light coconut milk and bring to a simmer.
4. Serve the curry over a bed of cooked brown rice.

Nutritional Information:

- Calories: 400
- Protein: 15g
- Carbohydrates: 60g
- Fiber: 12g
- Sugars: 6g
- Fat: 10g
- Saturated Fat: 5g
- Cholesterol: 0mg
- Sodium: 500mg

10. Salmon and Avocado Salad with Lemon-Dill Dressing

Prep Time: 15 minutes
Cooking Time: 15 minutes
Serving Size: 1
Ingredients:

- 4 ounces salmon fillet

- 1/2 avocado, sliced
- 1 cup mixed salad greens
- 1/4 cup cherry tomatoes, halved
- 1 tablespoon olive oil
- 1 tablespoon lemon juice
- 1 teaspoon fresh dill, chopped
- Salt and pepper to taste

Instructions:

1. Season salmon fillet with salt and pepper. Grill or bake until cooked through.

2. In a bowl, combine mixed salad greens, cherry tomatoes, and avocado slices.

3. Whisk together olive oil, lemon juice, and fresh dill to create the dressing.

4. Top the salad with grilled salmon and drizzle the lemon-dill dressing.

Nutritional Information:

- Calories: 420
- Protein: 30g
- Carbohydrates: 15g
- Fiber: 7g
- Sugars: 3g
- Fat: 30g
- Saturated Fat: 5g
- Cholesterol: 80mg

- Sodium: 400mg

11. Quinoa and Vegetable Stuffed Peppers

Prep Time: 25 minutes
Cooking Time: 30 minutes
Serving Size: 1
Ingredients:

- 1/2 cup quinoa, cooked

- 2 bell peppers, halved and seeds removed

- 1/2 cup black beans, cooked

- 1/2 cup corn kernels

- 1/4 cup red onion, finely chopped

- 1/2 cup diced tomatoes

- 1/2 teaspoon cumin

- 1/2 teaspoon chili powder

- Salt and pepper to taste

- 1/4 cup shredded cheddar cheese

Instructions:

1. Preheat the oven to 375°F (190°C).

2. In a bowl, mix cooked quinoa, black beans, corn, red onion, diced tomatoes, cumin, chili powder, salt, and pepper.

3. Spoon the mixture into halved bell peppers.

4. Sprinkle shredded cheddar cheese over the stuffed peppers.

5. Bake for 30 minutes or until peppers are tender.

Nutritional Information:

- Calories: 380

- Protein: 18g

- Carbohydrates: 55g

- Fiber: 12g

- Sugars: 6g

- Fat: 12g

- Saturated Fat: 5g

- Cholesterol: 20mg

- Sodium: 400mg

12. Chicken and Broccoli Quinoa Bowl

Prep Time: 20 minutes
Cooking Time: 20 minutes
Serving Size: 1
Ingredients:

- 4 ounces chicken breast, cooked and sliced

- 1/2 cup quinoa, cooked

- 1 cup broccoli florets

- 1/4 cup carrots, julienned

- 1 tablespoon low-sodium soy sauce

- 1 tablespoon hoisin sauce

- 1/2 teaspoon ginger, minced

- 1/2 teaspoon garlic, minced

- 1 tablespoon sesame seeds

Instructions:

1. In a pan, stir-fry broccoli and carrots until tender-crisp.

2. Add cooked and sliced chicken to the pan.

3. In a small bowl, mix soy sauce, hoisin sauce, ginger, and garlic. Pour over the chicken and vegetables.

4. Serve over a bed of cooked quinoa and sprinkle sesame seeds.

Nutritional Information:

- Calories: 420

- Protein: 30g

- Carbohydrates: 55g

- Fiber: 8g

- Sugars: 3g

- Fat: 12g

- Saturated Fat: 2.5g

- Cholesterol: 80mg

- Sodium: 600mg

13. Vegetable and Tofu Stir-Fry with Brown Rice

Prep Time: 20 minutes
Cooking Time: 15 minutes
Serving Size: 1
Ingredients:

- 1/2 cup extra-firm tofu, cubed

- 1 cup mixed stir-fry vegetables (broccoli, carrots, snap peas)

- 1 cup cooked brown rice

- 1 tablespoon low-sodium soy sauce

- 1 tablespoon hoisin sauce

- 1 teaspoon sesame oil
- 1/2 teaspoon garlic, minced
- 1/2 teaspoon ginger, minced

Instructions:

1. Press tofu to remove excess water and cut into cubes.
2. In a wok or skillet, stir-fry tofu until golden brown. Set aside.
3. Stir-fry mixed vegetables until tender-crisp.
4. Add cooked brown rice and tofu to the wok.
5. In a small bowl, mix soy sauce, hoisin sauce, sesame oil, garlic, and ginger. Pour over the mixture and toss until well combined.

Nutritional Information:

- Calories: 400
- Protein: 18g
- Carbohydrates: 55g
- Fiber: 8g
- Sugars: 3g
- Fat: 12g
- Saturated Fat: 2g
- Cholesterol: 0mg
- Sodium: 600mg

14. Greek Turkey Burger with Sweet Potato Wedges

Prep Time: 20 minutes
Cooking Time: 25 minutes
Serving Size: 1
Ingredients:

- 4 ounces lean ground turkey
- 1 whole-grain burger bun
- 1/4 cup cucumber, sliced
- 1/4 cup cherry tomatoes, halved
- 2 tablespoons feta cheese, crumbled
- 1 tablespoon Greek yogurt
- 1 sweet potato, cut into wedges
- 1 tablespoon olive oil
- 1/2 teaspoon dried oregano
- Salt and pepper to taste

Instructions:

1. Preheat the oven to 400°F (200°C).

2. Toss sweet potato wedges with olive oil, dried oregano, salt, and pepper. Roast for 20-25 minutes or until golden brown.

3. Season ground turkey with salt and pepper, then shape into a patty.

4. Grill or pan-fry the turkey burger until fully cooked.

5. Assemble the burger with cucumber slices, cherry tomatoes, feta cheese, and a dollop of Greek yogurt. Serve with sweet potato wedges.

Nutritional Information:

- Calories: 480
- Protein: 25g
- Carbohydrates: 55g
- Fiber: 8g
- Sugars: 8g
- Fat: 18g
- Saturated Fat: 5g
- Cholesterol: 60mg
- Sodium: 550mg

15. Sesame Ginger Salmon with Broccoli and Quinoa

Prep Time: 20 minutes
Cooking Time: 20 minutes
Serving Size: 1
Ingredients:

- 4 ounces salmon fillet
- 1/2 cup quinoa, cooked
- 1 cup broccoli florets
- 1 tablespoon low-sodium soy sauce
- 1 tablespoon rice vinegar
- 1 teaspoon sesame oil
- 1/2 teaspoon ginger, minced
- 1 clove garlic, minced

- Sesame seeds for garnish

Instructions:

1. Preheat the oven to 400°F (200°C).

2. Place salmon fillet on a baking sheet and surround with broccoli florets.

3. In a small bowl, whisk together soy sauce, rice vinegar, sesame oil, ginger, and garlic.

4. Brush the salmon with the sauce and drizzle the remaining sauce over the broccoli.

5. Bake for 15-20 minutes or until salmon is cooked through.

6. Serve over a bed of cooked quinoa and garnish with sesame seeds.

Nutritional Information:

- Calories: 450
- Protein: 30g
- Carbohydrates: 40g
- Fiber: 6g
- Sugars: 3g
- Fat: 20g
- Saturated Fat: 3.5g
- Cholesterol: 80mg
- Sodium: 500mg

16. Chickpea and Spinach Curry with Brown Rice

Prep Time: 20 minutes
Cooking Time: 25 minutes
Serving Size: 1
Ingredients:

- 1/2 cup canned chickpeas, drained and rinsed

- 1 cup spinach leaves

- 1/2 cup tomatoes, diced

- 1/4 cup red onion, finely chopped

- 1/2 cup light coconut milk

- 1 tablespoon curry powder

- 1/2 teaspoon turmeric

- 1/2 teaspoon cumin

- Salt and pepper to taste

- 1 cup cooked brown rice

Instructions:

1. In a pan, sauté red onion until softened.

2. Add chickpeas, tomatoes, curry powder, turmeric, cumin, salt, and pepper. Cook for 5 minutes.

3. Pour in light coconut milk and bring to a simmer.

4. Add spinach and cook until wilted.

5. Serve the curry over a bed of cooked brown rice.

Nutritional Information:

- Calories: 400

- Protein: 15g

- Carbohydrates: 60g

- Fiber: 12g

- Sugars: 6g

- Fat: 10g

- Saturated Fat: 5g

- Cholesterol: 0mg

- Sodium: 500mg

17. Teriyaki Tofu and Vegetable Skewers with Brown Rice

Prep Time: 20 minutes
Cooking Time: 15 minutes
Serving Size: 1
Ingredients:

- 1/2 cup extra-firm tofu, cubed

- 1 cup mixed vegetables (bell peppers, zucchini, mushrooms)

- 1/2 cup pineapple chunks

- 1/4 cup teriyaki sauce (low sodium)

- 1 cup cooked brown rice

- Sesame seeds for garnish

Instructions:

1. In a bowl, marinate tofu, mixed vegetables, and pineapple chunks in teriyaki sauce.

2. Thread tofu, vegetables, and pineapple onto skewers.

3. Grill or broil for 10-15 minutes, turning occasionally, until vegetables are tender.

4. Serve over a bed of cooked brown rice and sprinkle with sesame seeds.

Nutritional Information:

- Calories: 420

- Protein: 15g

- Carbohydrates: 65g

- Fiber: 8g

- Sugars: 12g

- Fat: 10g

- Saturated Fat: 1.5g

- Cholesterol: 0mg

- Sodium: 600mg

18. Quinoa and Black Bean Bowl with Avocado Salsa

Prep Time: 15 minutes
Cooking Time: 15 minutes
Serving Size: 1
Ingredients:

- 1/2 cup quinoa, cooked

- 1/2 cup black beans, cooked

- 1/4 cup corn kernels

- 1/4 cup red bell pepper, diced

- 1/4 cup cherry tomatoes, halved

- 1/2 avocado, diced

- 1 tablespoon cilantro, chopped

- 1 tablespoon lime juice

- Salt and pepper to taste

Instructions:

1. In a bowl, combine quinoa, black beans, corn, red bell pepper, and cherry tomatoes.

2. In a separate bowl, mix diced avocado, cilantro, lime juice, salt, and pepper to create the salsa.

3. Spoon the quinoa and black bean mixture into a bowl and top with avocado salsa.

Nutritional Information:

- Calories: 380

- Protein: 15g

- Carbohydrates: 55g

- Fiber: 12g

- Sugars: 5g

- Fat: 15g

- Saturated Fat: 2g

- Cholesterol: 0mg

- Sodium: 300mg

19. Vegetarian Fajita Bowl with Cauliflower Rice

Prep Time: 20 minutes
Cooking Time: 15 minutes
Serving Size: 1
Ingredients:

- 1/2 cup cauliflower rice, cooked
- 1/2 cup black beans, cooked
- 1/4 cup bell peppers, sliced
- 1/4 cup red onion, sliced
- 1/2 cup cherry tomatoes, halved
- 1/4 cup corn kernels
- 1/2 avocado, sliced
- 1 tablespoon olive oil
- 1 teaspoon taco seasoning
- Fresh cilantro for garnish

Instructions:

1. In a skillet, sauté bell peppers, red onion, cherry tomatoes, and corn in olive oil until tender.

2. Stir in black beans and taco seasoning, cooking for an additional 3-5 minutes.

3. Serve the fajita mixture over a bed of cooked cauliflower rice.

4. Top with sliced avocado and garnish with fresh cilantro.

Nutritional Information:

- Calories: 400

- Protein: 15g

- Carbohydrates: 60g

- Fiber: 15g

- Sugars: 8g

- Fat: 15g

- Saturated Fat: 2g

- Cholesterol: 0mg

- Sodium: 350mg

20. Mango Chicken Lettuce Wraps

Prep Time: 20 minutes
Cooking Time: 15 minutes
Serving Size: 1
Ingredients:

- 4 ounces chicken breast, cooked and shredded

- 1/2 mango, diced

- 1/4 cup red bell pepper, diced

- 2 tablespoons red onion, finely chopped

- 1 tablespoon cilantro, chopped

- 1 tablespoon lime juice

- Lettuce leaves for wrapping

Instructions:

1. In a bowl, combine shredded chicken, diced mango, red bell pepper, red onion, cilantro, and lime juice.

2. Mix until well combined.

3. Spoon the mixture onto lettuce leaves to create wraps.

Nutritional Information:

- Calories: 380
- Protein: 30g
- Carbohydrates: 40g
- Fiber: 6g
- Sugars: 18g
- Fat: 12g
- Saturated Fat: 2.5g
- Cholesterol: 80mg
- Sodium: 350mg

CHAPTER 7: SNACKS RECIPES

1. Greek Yogurt Parfait with Berries

Prep Time: 5 minutes

Serving Size: 1

Ingredients:

- 1/2 cup Greek yogurt

- 1/4 cup blueberries

- 1/4 cup strawberries, sliced

- 1 tablespoon honey

- 1 tablespoon chopped nuts (almonds or walnuts)

Instructions:

1. In a glass, layer Greek yogurt, blueberries, and sliced strawberries.

2. Drizzle honey over the layers.

3. Top with chopped nuts.

Nutritional Information:

- Calories: 200

- Protein: 15g

- Carbohydrates: 25g

- Fiber: 4g

- Sugars: 18g

- Fat: 8g

- Saturated Fat: 1g

- Cholesterol: 10mg

- Sodium: 30mg

2. Cucumber and Hummus Bites

Prep Time: 10 minutes

Serving Size: 1

Ingredients:

- 1 cucumber, sliced

- 2 tablespoons hummus

- Cherry tomatoes for garnish

- Fresh parsley for garnish

Instructions:

1. Top each cucumber slice with a small dollop of hummus.

2. Garnish with a cherry tomato and fresh parsley.

Nutritional Information:

- Calories: 50

- Protein: 2g

- Carbohydrates: 7g

- Fiber: 2g

- Sugars: 2g

- Fat: 2g

- Saturated Fat: 0g

- Cholesterol: 0mg

- Sodium: 70mg

3. Almond Butter Banana Wrap

Prep Time: 5 minutes

Serving Size: 1

Ingredients:

- 1 whole-grain tortilla

- 1 tablespoon almond butter

- 1 banana, sliced

Instructions:

1. Spread almond butter evenly over the tortilla.

2. Place banana slices in the center.

3. Roll the tortilla into a wrap.

Nutritional Information:

- Calories: 280

- Protein: 7g

- Carbohydrates: 45g

- Fiber: 6g

- Sugars: 15g

- Fat: 10g

- Saturated Fat: 1g

- Cholesterol: 0mg

- Sodium: 150mg

4. Caprese Skewers

Prep Time: 10 minutes

Serving Size: 1

Ingredients:

- Fresh mozzarella balls

- Cherry tomatoes

- Basil leaves

- Balsamic glaze for drizzling

Instructions:

1. Thread a mozzarella ball, a folded basil leaf, and a cherry tomato onto small skewers.

2. Arrange on a plate and drizzle with balsamic glaze.

Nutritional Information:

- Calories: 120

- Protein: 7g

- Carbohydrates: 5g

- Fiber: 1g

- Sugars: 3g

- Fat: 8g

- Saturated Fat: 5g

- Cholesterol: 30mg

- Sodium: 90mg

5. Apple Slices with Peanut Butter

Prep Time: 5 minutes

Serving Size: 1

Ingredients:

- 1 apple, sliced

- 2 tablespoons peanut butter

- Cinnamon for sprinkling (optional)

Instructions:

1. Spread peanut butter over apple slices.

2. Sprinkle with cinnamon if desired.

Nutritional Information:

- Calories: 220

- Protein: 6g

- Carbohydrates: 25g

- Fiber: 5g

- Sugars: 18g

- Fat: 12g

- Saturated Fat: 2g

- Cholesterol: 0mg

- Sodium: 90mg

6. Vegetable Sticks with Guacamole

Prep Time: 15 minutes
Serving Size: 1
Ingredients:

- Carrot and cucumber sticks

- 1/2 avocado, mashed

- 1 tablespoon lime juice

- Salt and pepper to taste

Instructions:

1. Mix mashed avocado with lime juice, salt, and pepper.

2. Serve with carrot and cucumber sticks.

Nutritional Information:

- Calories: 150

- Protein: 3g

- Carbohydrates: 12g

- Fiber: 7g

- Sugars: 3g

- Fat: 11g

- Saturated Fat: 2g

- Cholesterol: 0mg

- Sodium: 20mg

7. Chia Seed Pudding with Berries

Prep Time: 5 minutes (plus chilling time)

Serving Size: 1

Ingredients:

- 2 tablespoons chia seeds

- 1/2 cup almond milk

- 1/4 teaspoon vanilla extract

- Mixed berries for topping

Instructions:

1. Mix chia seeds, almond milk, and vanilla extract in a jar. Stir well.

2. Refrigerate for a few hours or overnight.

3. Top with mixed berries before serving.

Nutritional Information:

- Calories: 180

- Protein: 4g

- Carbohydrates: 20g

- Fiber: 10g

- Sugars: 5g

- Fat: 9g

- Saturated Fat: 1g

- Cholesterol: 0mg

- Sodium: 60mg

8. Hard-Boiled Egg and Avocado Slices

Prep Time: 15 minutes

Serving Size: 1

Ingredients:

- 1 hard-boiled egg, sliced

- 1/2 avocado, sliced

- Everything bagel seasoning for sprinkling

Instructions:

1. Arrange hard-boiled egg and avocado slices on a plate.

2. Sprinkle with everything bagel seasoning.

Nutritional Information:

- Calories: 210

- Protein: 10g

- Carbohydrates: 10g

- Fiber: 7g

- Sugars: 1g

- Fat: 15g

- Saturated Fat: 3.5g

- Cholesterol: 190mg

- Sodium: 140mg

9. Trail Mix with Nuts and Dried Fruit

Prep Time: 5 minutes

Serving Size: 1

Ingredients:

- 1/4 cup mixed nuts (almonds, walnuts, pistachios)

- 2 tablespoons dried cranberries

- 1 tablespoon dark chocolate chips

Instructions:

1. Mix nuts, dried cranberries, and dark chocolate chips in a bowl.

2. Portion into snack-sized servings.

Nutritional Information:

- Calories: 200

- Protein: 5g

- Carbohydrates: 15g

- Fiber: 3g

- Sugars: 9g

- Fat: 15g

- Saturated Fat: 2.5g

- Cholesterol: 0mg

- Sodium: 0mg

10. Rice Cake with Cottage Cheese and Pineapple

Prep Time: 5 minutes

Serving Size: 1

Ingredients:

- 1 rice cake

- 1/2 cup low-fat cottage cheese

- 1/4 cup pineapple chunks

Instructions:

1. Spread cottage cheese over the rice cake.

2. Top with pineapple chunks.

Nutritional Information:

- Calories: 180

- Protein: 15g

- Carbohydrates: 25g

- Fiber: 2g

- Sugars: 10g

- Fat: 2g

- Saturated Fat: 1g

- Cholesterol: 10mg

- Sodium: 330mg

11. Sliced Bell Peppers with Hummus

Prep Time: 10 minutes

Serving Size: 1

Ingredients:

- Assorted bell peppers, sliced

- 2 tablespoons hummus

Instructions:

1. Arrange sliced bell peppers on a plate.

2. Serve with hummus for dipping.

Nutritional Information:

- Calories: 70

- Protein: 2g

- Carbohydrates: 10g

- Fiber: 3g

- Sugars: 6g

- Fat: 3g

- Saturated Fat: 0g

- Cholesterol: 0mg

- Sodium: 150mg

12. Cheese and Whole Grain Crackers

Prep Time: 5 minutes

Serving Size: 1

Ingredients:

- 1 ounce cheese (cheddar, mozzarella)

- 1 serving whole-grain crackers

Instructions:

1. Arrange cheese and whole-grain crackers on a plate.

Nutritional Information:

- Calories: 180

- Protein: 8g

- Carbohydrates: 15g

- Fiber: 3g

- Sugars: 0g

- Fat: 10g

- Saturated Fat: 6g

- Cholesterol: 30mg

- Sodium: 230mg

13. Edamame and Sea Salt

Prep Time: 5 minutes

Serving Size: 1

Ingredients:

- 1 cup edamame, steamed
- Sea salt for sprinkling

Instructions:

1. Steam edamame according to package instructions.
2. Sprinkle with sea salt.

Nutritional Information:

- Calories: 150
- Protein: 13g
- Carbohydrates: 11g
- Fiber: 6g
- Sugars: 2g
- Fat: 8g
- Saturated Fat: 1g
- Cholesterol: 0mg
- Sodium: 5mg

14. Yogurt-Covered Strawberries

Prep Time: 10 minutes

Serving Size: 1

Ingredients:

- 1/2 cup strawberries, whole or halved

- 2 tablespoons yogurt (Greek or regular)

Instructions:

1. Dip each strawberry into yogurt until coated.

2. Place on a tray and freeze until yogurt is set.

Nutritional Information:

- Calories: 90

- Protein: 3g

- Carbohydrates: 15g

- Fiber: 2g

- Sugars: 10g

- Fat: 2g

- Saturated Fat: 1g

- Cholesterol: 5mg

- Sodium: 20mg

15. Turkey and Cheese Roll-Ups

Prep Time: 10 minutes

Serving Size: 1

Ingredients:

- 4 slices turkey breast

- 2 slices low-fat cheese

- Mustard for spreading

Instructions:

1. Spread mustard on each turkey slice.

2. Place a slice of cheese on top and roll up.

Nutritional Information:

- Calories: 160

- Protein: 18g

- Carbohydrates: 2g

- Fiber: 0g

- Sugars: 1g

- Fat: 9g

- Saturated Fat: 4g

- Cholesterol: 40mg

- Sodium: 550mg

16. Pita Bread with Hummus and Sliced Olives

Prep Time: 8 minutes

Serving Size: 1

Ingredients:

- 1 whole-grain pita bread

- 2 tablespoons hummus

- Sliced olives for topping

Instructions:

1. Warm the pita bread.

2. Spread hummus over the pita and top with sliced olives.

Nutritional Information:

- Calories: 180

- Protein: 6g

- Carbohydrates: 25g

- Fiber: 5g

- Sugars: 1g

- Fat: 7g

- Saturated Fat: 1g

- Cholesterol: 0mg

- Sodium: 300mg

17. Homemade Popcorn with Parmesan

Prep Time: 5 minutes

Cooking Time: 5 minutes

Serving Size: 1

Ingredients:

- 1/2 cup popcorn kernels

- 2 tablespoons grated Parmesan cheese

- 1 tablespoon olive oil

- Salt to taste

Instructions:

1. Pop the popcorn kernels.

2. Drizzle with olive oil, sprinkle Parmesan and salt. Toss to coat.

Nutritional Information:

- Calories: 200

- Protein: 5g

- Carbohydrates: 25g

- Fiber: 5g

- Sugars: 0g

- Fat: 10g

- Saturated Fat: 2g

- Cholesterol: 5mg

- Sodium: 200mg

18. Mango Salsa with Baked Tortilla Chips

Prep Time: 15 minutes

Cooking Time: 10 minutes

Serving Size: 1

Ingredients:

- 1 mango, diced

- 1/4 cup red onion, finely chopped

- 1/4 cup cilantro, chopped

- 1 tablespoon lime juice

- Whole-grain tortilla chips for serving

Instructions:

1. Mix diced mango, red onion, cilantro, and lime juice in a bowl.

2. Bake whole-grain tortilla chips until crispy.

Nutritional Information:

- Calories: 180

- Protein: 2g

- Carbohydrates: 40g

- Fiber: 5g

- Sugars: 25g

- Fat: 3g

- Saturated Fat: 0g

- Cholesterol: 0mg

- Sodium: 120mg

19. Oat and Nut Energy Balls

Prep Time: 15 minutes

Serving Size: 1

Ingredients:

- 1 cup rolled oats

- 1/2 cup nut butter

- 1/4 cup honey

- 1/4 cup chopped nuts (almonds, walnuts)

- Dark chocolate chips for rolling

Instructions:

1. Mix rolled oats, nut butter, honey, and chopped nuts in a bowl.

2. Form into small balls and roll in dark chocolate chips.

Nutritional Information:

- Calories: 180

- Protein: 6g

- Carbohydrates: 20g

- Fiber: 3g

- Sugars: 9g

- Fat: 10g

- Saturated Fat: 2g

- Cholesterol: 0mg

- Sodium: 20mg

20. Baked Sweet Potato Chips

Prep Time: 15 minutes

Cooking Time: 20 minutes

Serving Size: 1

Ingredients:

- 1 sweet potato, thinly sliced

- 1 tablespoon olive oil

- Paprika for sprinkling

- Sea salt to taste

Instructions:

1. Preheat the oven to 400°F (200°C).

2. Toss sweet potato slices in olive oil, paprika, and sea salt.

3. Bake until crispy.

Nutritional Information:

- Calories: 150

- Protein: 2g

- Carbohydrates: 25g

- Fiber: 4g

- Sugars: 6g

- Fat: 5g

- Saturated Fat: 0.5g

- Cholesterol: 0mg

- Sodium: 150mg

CHAPTER 8: DESSERT RECIPES

1. Chia Seed Pudding with Mixed Berries

Prep Time: 5 minutes (plus chilling time)

Cooking Time: 0 minutes

Serving Size: 1

Ingredients:

- 2 tablespoons chia seeds

- 1/2 cup unsweetened almond milk

- 1/4 teaspoon vanilla extract

- Mixed berries for topping

Instructions:

1. Mix chia seeds, almond milk, and vanilla extract in a jar. Stir well.

2. Refrigerate for a few hours or overnight.

3. Top with mixed berries before serving.

Nutritional Information:

- Calories: 180

- Protein: 4g

- Carbohydrates: 20g

- Fiber: 10g

- Sugars: 5g

- Fat: 9g

- Saturated Fat: 1g

- Cholesterol: 0mg

- Sodium: 60mg

2. Baked Apples with Cinnamon and Walnuts

Prep Time: 10 minutes

Cooking Time: 30 minutes

Serving Size: 1

Ingredients:

- 1 apple, cored and sliced

- 1/2 teaspoon cinnamon

- 1 tablespoon chopped walnuts

- 1 teaspoon honey

Instructions:

1. Preheat the oven to 375°F (190°C).

2. Place apple slices in a baking dish and sprinkle with cinnamon.

3. Top with chopped walnuts and drizzle with honey.

4. Bake for 30 minutes or until apples are tender.

Nutritional Information:

- Calories: 150

- Protein: 1g

- Carbohydrates: 30g

- Fiber: 5g

- Sugars: 20g

- Fat: 4g

- Saturated Fat: 0.5g

- Cholesterol: 0mg

- Sodium: 0mg

3. Greek Yogurt and Berry Parfait

Prep Time: 5 minutes

Cooking Time: 0 minutes

Serving Size: 1

Ingredients:

- 1/2 cup Greek yogurt

- 1/4 cup mixed berries

- 1 tablespoon honey

- 1 tablespoon granola (optional)

Instructions:

1. In a glass, layer Greek yogurt and mixed berries.

2. Drizzle honey over the layers.

3. Top with granola if desired.

Nutritional Information:

- Calories: 200

- Protein: 15g

- Carbohydrates: 25g

- Fiber: 4g

- Sugars: 18g

- Fat: 8g

- Saturated Fat: 1g

- Cholesterol: 10mg

- Sodium: 30mg

4. Avocado Chocolate Mousse

Prep Time: 10 minutes

Cooking Time: 0 minutes

Serving Size: 1

Ingredients:

- 1 ripe avocado

- 2 tablespoons unsweetened cocoa powder

- 2 tablespoons maple syrup

- 1/2 teaspoon vanilla extract

- Pinch of salt

Instructions:

1. In a blender, combine avocado, cocoa powder, maple syrup, vanilla extract, and a pinch of salt.

2. Blend until smooth and creamy.

3. Chill before serving.

Nutritional Information:

- Calories: 250

- Protein: 3g

- Carbohydrates: 30g

- Fiber: 8g

- Sugars: 18g

- Fat: 15g

- Saturated Fat: 2g

- Cholesterol: 0mg

- Sodium: 10mg

5. Coconut Almond Balls

Prep Time: 15 minutes

Cooking Time: 0 minutes

Serving Size: 1

Ingredients:

- 1 cup shredded coconut

- 1/2 cup almond flour

- 2 tablespoons coconut oil, melted

- 1 tablespoon honey

- 1/2 teaspoon almond extract

Instructions:

1. In a bowl, mix shredded coconut, almond flour, melted coconut oil, honey, and almond extract.

2. Shape into balls and refrigerate until firm.

Nutritional Information:

- Calories: 180

- Protein: 3g

- Carbohydrates: 8g

- Fiber: 5g

- Sugars: 4g

- Fat: 15g

- Saturated Fat: 10g

- Cholesterol: 0mg

- Sodium: 5mg

6. Banana Oatmeal Cookies

Prep Time: 10 minutes

Cooking Time: 15 minutes

Serving Size: 1

Ingredients:

- 1 ripe banana, mashed

- 1 cup rolled oats

- 1/4 cup chopped nuts (walnuts or almonds)

- 1/4 cup raisins

- 1/2 teaspoon vanilla extract

Instructions:

1. Preheat the oven to 350°F (175°C).

2. In a bowl, combine mashed banana, rolled oats, chopped nuts, raisins, and vanilla extract.

3. Drop spoonfuls onto a baking sheet and bake for 15 minutes.

Nutritional Information:

- Calories: 180

- Protein: 4g

- Carbohydrates: 30g

- Fiber: 4g

- Sugars: 12g

- Fat: 6g

- Saturated Fat: 1g

- Cholesterol: 0mg

- Sodium: 0mg

7. Pumpkin Spice Muffins

Prep Time: 15 minutes

Cooking Time: 20 minutes

Serving Size: 1

Ingredients:

- 1 cup canned pumpkin puree

- 1/2 cup almond flour

- 1/2 cup coconut flour

- 1/4 cup coconut oil, melted

- 1/4 cup maple syrup

- 2 eggs

- 1 teaspoon baking powder

- 1/2 teaspoon cinnamon

- 1/4 teaspoon nutmeg

- Pinch of salt

Instructions:

1. Preheat the oven to 350°F (175°C).

2. In a bowl, mix pumpkin puree, almond flour, coconut flour, melted coconut oil, maple syrup, eggs, baking powder, cinnamon, nutmeg, and a pinch of salt.

3. Spoon into muffin cups and bake for 20 minutes.

Nutritional Information:

- Calories: 180

- Protein: 5g

- Carbohydrates: 20g

- Fiber: 5g

- Sugars: 8g

- Fat: 10g

- Saturated Fat: 7g

- Cholesterol: 40mg

- Sodium: 50mg

8. Berry and Almond Crisp

Prep Time: 15 minutes
Cooking Time: 30 minutes
Serving Size: 1
Ingredients:

- 1 cup mixed berries (blueberries, strawberries, raspberries)

- 2 tablespoons almond flour

- 1 tablespoon maple syrup

- 1/4 cup rolled oats

- 1 tablespoon sliced almonds

Instructions:

1. Preheat the oven to 375°F (190°C).

2. In a bowl, mix mixed berries, almond flour, maple syrup, rolled oats, and sliced almonds.

3. Transfer to a baking dish and bake for 30 minutes.

Nutritional Information:

- Calories: 200

- Protein: 4g

- Carbohydrates: 30g

- Fiber: 5g

- Sugars: 15g

- Fat: 8g

- Saturated Fat: 0.5g

- Cholesterol: 0mg

- Sodium: 5mg

9. Chocolate Avocado Mousse

Prep Time: 10 minutes

Cooking Time: 0 minutes

Serving Size: 1

Ingredients:

- 1 ripe avocado

- 2 tablespoons unsweetened cocoa powder

- 3 tablespoons honey

- 1/2 teaspoon vanilla extract

- Pinch of salt

Instructions:

1. In a blender, combine ripe avocado, cocoa powder, honey, vanilla extract, and a pinch of salt.

2. Blend until smooth.

3. Chill before serving.

Nutritional Information:

- Calories: 250

- Protein: 3g

- Carbohydrates: 30g

- Fiber: 8g

- Sugars: 20g

- Fat: 15g

- Saturated Fat: 2g

- Cholesterol: 0mg

- Sodium: 10mg

10. Walnut and Banana Bread

Prep Time: 15 minutes

Cooking Time: 45 minutes

Serving Size: 1 slice

Ingredients:

- 1 cup mashed ripe bananas

- 1/4 cup coconut oil, melted

- 1/4 cup maple syrup

- 2 eggs

- 1 teaspoon vanilla extract

- 1 3/4 cups almond flour

- 1/2 teaspoon baking soda

- 1/4 teaspoon salt

- 1/2 cup chopped walnuts

Instructions:

1. Preheat the oven to 350°F (175°C).

2. In a bowl, mix mashed bananas, melted coconut oil, maple syrup, eggs, and vanilla extract.

3. Add almond flour, baking soda, and salt. Mix until well combined.

4. Fold in chopped walnuts.

5. Pour into a greased loaf pan and bake for 45 minutes.

Nutritional Information:

- Calories: 220

- Protein: 6g

- Carbohydrates: 20g

- Fiber: 4g

- Sugars: 10g

- Fat: 15g

- Saturated Fat: 4g

- Cholesterol: 40mg

- Sodium: 150mg

11. Peach and Berry Sorbet

Prep Time: 10 minutes (plus freezing time)

Cooking Time: 0 minutes

Serving Size: 1

Ingredients:

- 1 cup frozen peaches

- 1/2 cup mixed berries

- 2 tablespoons honey

- 1/4 cup water

Instructions:

1. In a blender, combine frozen peaches, mixed berries, honey, and water.

2. Blend until smooth.

3. Pour into a container and freeze until firm.

Nutritional Information:

- Calories: 150

- Protein: 1g

- Carbohydrates: 40g

- Fiber: 5g

- Sugars: 30g

- Fat: 0g

- Saturated Fat: 0g

- Cholesterol: 0mg

- Sodium: 0mg

12. Cinnamon Baked Pears

Prep Time: 10 minutes

Cooking Time: 30 minutes

Serving Size: 1

Ingredients:

- 1 pear, halved and cored

- 1/2 teaspoon cinnamon

- 1 tablespoon chopped pecans

- 1 teaspoon honey

Instructions:

1. Preheat the oven to 375°F (190°C).

2. Place pear halves in a baking dish.

3. Sprinkle with cinnamon, chopped pecans, and drizzle with honey.

4. Bake for 30 minutes or until pears are tender.

Nutritional Information:

- Calories: 180

- Protein: 2g

- Carbohydrates: 30g

- Fiber: 6g

- Sugars: 18g

- Fat: 8g

- Saturated Fat: 0.5g

- Cholesterol: 0mg

- Sodium: 0mg

13. Blueberry Almond Crumble Bars

Prep Time: 15 minutes

Cooking Time: 30 minutes

Serving Size: 1 bar

Ingredients:

- 1 cup almond flour

- 1/4 cup coconut flour

- 1/4 cup coconut oil, melted

- 1/4 cup maple syrup

- 1/2 teaspoon almond extract

- 1 cup fresh blueberries

Instructions:

1. Preheat the oven to 350°F (175°C).

2. In a bowl, combine almond flour, coconut flour, melted coconut oil, maple syrup, and almond extract.

3. Press half of the mixture into a baking pan.

4. Sprinkle fresh blueberries over the crust.

5. Crumble the remaining mixture on top.

6. Bake for 30 minutes or until golden.

Nutritional Information:

- Calories: 220

- Protein: 5g

- Carbohydrates: 20g

- Fiber: 5g

- Sugars: 10g

- Fat: 15g

- Saturated Fat: 7g

- Cholesterol: 0mg

- Sodium: 5mg

14. Cocoa Dusted Almonds

Prep Time: 5 minutes

Cooking Time: 10 minutes

Serving Size: 1

Ingredients:

- 1 cup raw almonds

- 1 tablespoon unsweetened cocoa powder

- 1 tablespoon honey

- Pinch of sea salt

Instructions:

1. Preheat the oven to 350°F (175°C).

2. In a bowl, toss raw almonds with cocoa powder, honey, and a pinch of sea salt.

3. Spread on a baking sheet and bake for 10 minutes.

Nutritional Information:

- Calories: 200

- Protein: 7g

- Carbohydrates: 15g

- Fiber: 5g

- Sugars: 7g

- Fat: 15g

- Saturated Fat: 1g

- Cholesterol: 0mg

- Sodium: 0mg

15. Mango Coconut Rice Pudding

Prep Time: 10 minutes

Cooking Time: 25 minutes

Serving Size: 1

Ingredients:

- 1/2 cup cooked brown rice

- 1/2 cup coconut milk

- 1/4 cup diced mango

- 1 tablespoon shredded coconut

- 1 tablespoon agave syrup

Instructions:

1. In a saucepan, combine cooked brown rice and coconut milk. Simmer for 20 minutes.

2. Stir in diced mango and shredded coconut.

3. Sweeten with agave syrup.

Nutritional Information:

- Calories: 220

- Protein: 3g

- Carbohydrates: 35g

- Fiber: 4g

- Sugars: 12g

- Fat: 8g

- Saturated Fat: 6g

- Cholesterol: 0mg

- Sodium: 10mg

16. Pistachio Date Bites

Prep Time: 15 minutes

Cooking Time: 0 minutes

Serving Size: 1

Ingredients:

- 1 cup pitted dates

- 1/2 cup shelled pistachios

- 1/4 cup unsweetened shredded coconut

Instructions:

1. In a food processor, blend pitted dates and shelled pistachios until a sticky dough forms.

2. Roll into bite-sized balls and coat with shredded coconut.

Nutritional Information:

- Calories: 180

- Protein: 3g

- Carbohydrates: 30g

- Fiber: 4g

- Sugars: 25g

- Fat: 8g

- Saturated Fat: 2g

- Cholesterol: 0mg

- Sodium: 5mg

17. Pomegranate and Walnut Salad

Prep Time: 10 minutes
Cooking Time: 0 minutes
Serving Size: 1
Ingredients:

- 1/2 cup pomegranate arils

- 2 tablespoons chopped walnuts

- 1 tablespoon honey

- 1 teaspoon lemon juice

Instructions:

1. In a bowl, mix pomegranate arils, chopped walnuts, honey, and lemon juice.

2. Toss until well combined.

Nutritional Information:

- Calories: 150

- Protein: 3g

- Carbohydrates: 20g

- Fiber: 4g

- Sugars: 14g

- Fat: 8g

- Saturated Fat: 0.5g

- Cholesterol: 0mg

- Sodium: 0mg

18. Cranberry Orange Quinoa Salad

Prep Time: 15 minutes

Cooking Time: 15 minutes

Serving Size: 1

Ingredients:

- 1/2 cup cooked quinoa

- 2 tablespoons dried cranberries

- 1 tablespoon chopped almonds

- 1 tablespoon orange zest

- 1 tablespoon orange juice

- 1 teaspoon maple syrup

Instructions:

1. In a bowl, combine cooked quinoa, dried cranberries, chopped almonds, orange zest, orange juice, and maple syrup.

2. Toss until well mixed.

Nutritional Information:

- Calories: 180

- Protein: 4g

- Carbohydrates: 30g

- Fiber: 3g

- Sugars: 8g

- Fat: 5g

- Saturated Fat: 0.5g

- Cholesterol: 0mg

- Sodium: 0mg

19. Apricot Almond Energy Bites

Prep Time: 15 minutes

Cooking Time: 0 minutes

Serving Size: 1

Ingredients:

- 1/2 cup dried apricots

- 1/2 cup almonds

- 1/4 cup rolled oats

- 1 tablespoon chia seeds

- 1 tablespoon honey

Instructions:

1. In a food processor, blend dried apricots, almonds, rolled oats, chia seeds, and honey until a sticky mixture forms.

2. Roll into bite-sized balls.

Nutritional Information:

- Calories: 180

- Protein: 4g

- Carbohydrates: 25g

- Fiber: 4g

- Sugars: 15g

- Fat: 9g

- Saturated Fat: 0.5g

- Cholesterol: 0mg

- Sodium: 0mg

20. Dark Chocolate-Covered Strawberries

Prep Time: 10 minutes

Cooking Time: 0 minutes

Serving Size: 2

Ingredients:

- 1/2 cup dark chocolate chips

- 1 cup strawberries, washed and dried

Instructions:

1. Melt dark chocolate chips in a microwave-safe bowl.

2. Dip each strawberry into melted chocolate, coating half of the strawberry.

3. Place on a tray and refrigerate until chocolate is set.

Nutritional Information:

- Calories: 200

- Protein: 2g

- Carbohydrates: 30g

- Fiber: 6g

- Sugars: 20g

- Fat: 10g

- Saturated Fat: 6g

- Cholesterol: 0mg

- Sodium: 0mg

CHAPTER 9: LIFESTYLE CHANGES AND EXERCISE

Incorporating Physical Activity into Daily Routine

Living with CKD Stage 3 and Diabetes Type 2 requires a holistic approach that goes beyond dietary considerations. Physical activity is a cornerstone of a healthy lifestyle and plays a pivotal role in managing these health conditions. Incorporating exercise into your daily routine can have profound benefits for both your physical and mental well-being.

The Role of Exercise in CKD and Diabetes Management

Regular physical activity has been shown to have numerous benefits for individuals with CKD and Diabetes Type 2. Exercise helps improve insulin sensitivity, making it easier for the body to regulate blood sugar levels. It also aids in weight management, which is crucial for individuals with diabetes and CKD, as excess weight can exacerbate these conditions.

In the case of CKD, exercise contributes to better cardiovascular health, which is often compromised in kidney disease. It helps regulate blood pressure, reduces the risk of cardiovascular events, and enhances overall circulation, promoting kidney function.

Moreover, engaging in regular exercise has positive effects on mental health. It reduces stress, anxiety, and depression, common concerns for those dealing with chronic health conditions. Establishing a routine that includes physical activity can provide a sense of accomplishment and boost mood, contributing to an improved quality of life.

Tailoring Exercise to Individual Needs

It's crucial to recognize that not all exercises are suitable for everyone, especially for seniors managing CKD Stage 3 and Diabetes Type 2. Before embarking on any exercise routine, consulting with healthcare professionals is essential. They can provide personalized recommendations based on individual health status, limitations, and specific needs.

Low-impact exercises, such as walking, swimming, or cycling, are generally well-tolerated and beneficial for individuals with CKD and diabetes. These activities are gentle on the joints, making them suitable for seniors. Resistance training can also be incorporated to improve muscle strength and support overall mobility.

Remember to start slowly and gradually increase the intensity and duration of your exercises. Listening to your body and adjusting your routine accordingly is key to a sustainable and enjoyable exercise regimen.

Chair Exercises for Seniors

For seniors managing CKD Stage 3 and Diabetes Type 2, incorporating physical activity doesn't always mean hitting the gym or engaging in high-impact workouts. Chair exercises offer a convenient and accessible alternative, allowing individuals to stay active while seated.

Benefits of Chair Exercises

Chair exercises provide a range of benefits, especially for seniors with mobility limitations. They enhance flexibility, strengthen muscles, and improve balance—all crucial aspects of maintaining overall physical function. These exercises can be tailored to individual fitness levels and adjusted to accommodate specific health concerns.

Seated Leg Lifts

Seated leg lifts are a simple yet effective exercise for seniors. While sitting in a sturdy chair, straighten one or both legs and hold in place for a few seconds. Lower the leg(s) back to the ground without letting the feet touch the floor. Repeat this movement for a set number of repetitions. This exercise helps strengthen the quadriceps and improves circulation.

Chair Squats

Chair squats are excellent for strengthening the lower body muscles, including the thighs and buttocks. Stand in front of a chair with feet shoulder-width apart. Lower the body into a sitting position without fully sitting down, then return to a standing position. Repeat for a set number of repetitions. This exercise promotes leg strength and functional mobility.

Seated Marching

Seated marching is a simple cardiovascular exercise that can be done while sitting in a chair. Lift one knee at a time toward the chest in a marching motion. Continue this movement for a set period, gradually increasing the duration as endurance improves. Seated marching helps elevate the heart rate and improve cardiovascular health.

Safety Considerations for Chair Exercises

While chair exercises are generally safe for seniors, certain precautions should be taken to ensure a positive and injury-free experience. It's important to use a stable chair without wheels and to perform these exercises on a non-slip surface.

Additionally, individuals should be aware of their own limitations and avoid overexertion. If there is any discomfort or pain during exercises, it's crucial to stop and consult with a healthcare professional. The goal is to engage in activities that promote well-being without causing harm.

Importance of Regular Movement

Living a sedentary lifestyle can have detrimental effects on overall health, particularly for seniors managing CKD Stage 3 and Diabetes Type 2. Incorporating regular movement into your daily routine is a fundamental aspect of maintaining physical and mental well-being.

Counteracting the Risks of Sedentary Behavior

Sitting for extended periods can contribute to various health risks, including increased blood pressure, impaired glucose metabolism, and weight gain. For individuals with diabetes and CKD, these risks can exacerbate existing health issues.

Regular movement, even in short intervals, helps counteract these risks. Simple activities such as stretching, standing up and walking around, or performing light exercises can have significant positive effects. These movements improve blood circulation, enhance joint flexibility, and contribute to better overall metabolic health.

Tips for Incorporating Movement into Daily Life

1. **Set Reminders:** Use alarms or smartphone reminders to prompt short breaks for movement throughout the day. This could involve standing up, stretching, or taking a short walk.

2. **Choose Active Hobbies:** Opt for hobbies that involve physical activity, such as gardening, dancing, or swimming. Engaging in activities you enjoy makes it more likely that you'll stick to them.

3. **Use Supportive Footwear:** Wearing comfortable and supportive footwear encourages movement. It makes walking and standing activities more enjoyable and reduces the risk of discomfort or injury.

4. **Break Up Sitting Time:** If your routine involves prolonged periods of sitting, break it up with short intervals of movement. Stand up, stretch, or take a brief walk every hour.

5. **Involve Family and Friends:** Make physical activity a social affair by involving family or friends. This could include taking walks together, participating in group exercises, or joining a dance class.

The Role of Movement in Mental Health

Regular movement not only benefits physical health but also plays a crucial role in maintaining mental well-being. Physical activity stimulates the release of endorphins, which are neurotransmitters that promote feelings of happiness and reduce the perception of pain. For individuals managing chronic health conditions, the positive impact on mental health is particularly significant.

CONCLUSION

As we conclude this journey through the "CKD Stage 3 and Diabetes Type 2 Cookbook for Seniors," I want to extend my heartfelt appreciation for joining me on this exploration of health, nutrition, and wellness tailored specifically for seniors navigating the challenges of chronic kidney disease (CKD) Stage 3 and Diabetes Type 2.

In the pages of this cookbook, we've embarked on a quest to create not just meals but experiences—culinary journeys designed to nourish the body, tantalize the taste buds, and foster a sense of well-being. Each recipe is a testament to the fusion of deliciousness and health-conscious choices, demonstrating that managing health conditions doesn't mean sacrificing the joy of savoring delectable flavors.

Our culinary adventure began with an insightful overview of CKD Stage 3 and Diabetes Type 2, offering a compass to navigate the complexities of these conditions. From understanding the intricacies of kidney health to unraveling the nuances of diabetes management, we set the stage for a holistic approach to senior health.

Moving forward, we delved into the nuances of dietary choices. In Chapter 1, we explored the art of balancing carbohydrates, proteins, and fats—a delicate dance that becomes even more crucial when faced with CKD Stage 3 and Diabetes Type 2. The chapter unveiled the importance of fiber in the diet, acting as a gentle guide toward better digestive health and blood sugar control. Simultaneously, we navigated the waters of sodium intake, recognizing the impact on kidney function and blood pressure.

Chapter 2 ushered us into the realm of monitoring and managing health. Regular checkups, blood sugar monitoring, understanding kidney function tests, and medication management became the pillars of a proactive and informed approach to health. Knowledge, after all, is a powerful ally on the journey toward well-being.

In Chapter 3, we ventured into the heart of the home—the kitchen. Smart cooking techniques for seniors, easy meal prep ideas, and the convenience of batch cooking were unveiled as invaluable tools to make the kitchen a sanctuary of health and flavor.

Our cookbook journey reached its pinnacle with a symphony of recipes designed to delight the palate while aligning with the dietary considerations of CKD Stage 3 and Diabetes Type 2. From breakfast to dinner, and every snack in between, these recipes were crafted with care and consideration, offering a tapestry of flavors that underscored the joy of mindful eating.

As we explored lifestyle changes and the importance of regular movement in Chapter 9, we emphasized the significance of a holistic approach to health. Physical activity, even in the form of chair exercises for seniors, emerged as a key player in enhancing both physical and mental well-being.

In this final reflection, I invite you to carry the essence of this cookbook into your daily life—a celebration of health, a commitment to mindful choices, and an embrace of the joy that arises when nourishing your body becomes a heartfelt ritual.

Remember, this cookbook is not just a collection of recipes; it's a companion on your journey toward a healthier and more vibrant life. May these pages continue to inspire and guide you as you savor the richness of each moment, one delicious and health-conscious bite at a time.

Thank you for entrusting me with a part of your culinary and wellness voyage. Here's to your health, happiness, and the countless flavors yet to be discovered on your unique path.

Made in the USA
Las Vegas, NV
16 February 2024

85879029R00105